Praise for *The Best Gluten-Free Family Cookbook* and *125 Best Gluten-Free Recipes*

"I recently attended a fabulous gluten-free workshop given by Donna and Heather. They spoke joyfully of the hours upon hours spent in their test kitchen finding the most delicious ways to incorporate nutritious flours into their recipes. Full of practical information in addition to the recipes, this cookbook can serve as an excellent resource for any GF home cook."

— Amy E. Pagano, MS, RD, Outpatient Nutritionist, University of Virginia Health System

"Thanks for the time and effort you've put into these cookbooks. I love cooking and baking and was 'thrown for a loop' when my daughter was diagnosed with celiac disease. Now I'm 'relearning' how to cook (I feel semi-panicky not having my old, trusted recipes to fall back on and haven't ventured far enough to try and make them over in a gluten-free variation), and your cookbooks are making that learning process enjoyable and not terrifying!"

— Shelley Conway, Newberry Springs, California

"I made your Strawberry Rhubarb Pie this weekend. It is so melt-in-the-mouth good! My husband, not a celiac, just can't get enough of it. It was the first of your recipes I attempted after hearing you speak at one of our meetings. I've had no failures, and everything is so tasty."

— Sheila Green, member, London Chapter, Canadian Celiac Association

"I called my neighbor over to taste the Mediterranean Pizza Squares since he's a chef at a health food store. He thought it was great, and his wife said it was the best pizza she had ever eaten!"

— Judy Hodges, Richmond, Virginia

"I have had the most success when using the Washburn and Butt cookbooks. I especially like their bread machine recipes — always tasty. Henk's Flax Bread tastes like whole wheat bread. I can't recommend this book enough for beginners. And besides the bread recipes, there are loads of recipes for all kinds of meals you can make for the entire family."

— R. Stanhope, Boston, Massachusetts

"I was absolutely delighted with the gluten-free Ciabatta recipe. For the first time since my diagnosis, I actually was able to have sandwiches for lunch — it was fabulous! I also made the gluten-free Greek Pasta Salad this week for lunch, and my officemate complained that it smelled 'too good.' Just want to give you a 'job well done.'"

— Rebecca Goyan, Kingston, Ontario

"How nice to be able to send chocolate chip cookies to a school bake sale. Or serve up pizza and chocolate cake for my 11-year-old daughter's birthday party. The gluten-eating family members are enjoying the GF foods as well, and don't even realize the difference until I tell them. Oh, and the pastry recipe! . . . Thanks so much for all the work that goes into creating, testing and retesting these recipes."

—Kae Moore, Port Hope, Ontario

"I just earned a blue ribbon (in the gluten-free muffin category) at our local fair with your Applesauce Raisin Muffin recipe."

— Cecelia Lane, Everett, Washington

"It's so joyful to see Connie enjoy an honest slice or two of buttered bread with a pot of tea . . . when she got diagnosed with celiac disease, it was a kind of a slow-motion crushing blow we thought we'd never get over . . . but now there's a semblance of normalcy, thanks to people like you two nice ladies."

— Michel Synnett, Picton, Ontario

"Your books saved my life. I love your Chocolate Chip Cookies; in fact, so do my kids — the cookies don't make it to the dish. I have to tell them, 'Slow down — they're the cookies Mommy can eat.' Your Pumpernickel Loaf is also great. I even used it to make bread crumbs. The Banana Nut Muffins help me get through breakfast and a late-night snack. Your Hamburger Buns are getting me through the summer. I'm grateful for your books and for the chance to say thank you for making my life not so sad."

— Jacqueline Braue, New York

"The Best Gluten-Free cookbooks contain a variety of whole-grain recipes that are much more nutritious than the standard rice flour recipes. The extensive tips and testing make these cookbooks appropriate for an individual without a lot of knowledge or skill."

— Wendy Busse, Dietitians of Canada newsletter

"Congratulations! Your book [125 Best Gluten-Free Recipes] has been nominated for the 2004 Cuisine Canada/University of Guelph National Culinary Book Awards. Your book will be placed in the University of Guelph Library's archival cookbook collection."

— Jo Marie Powers, Chair, Culinary Book Awards, Cuisine Canada

"Tim Hortons can't touch me when it comes to making muffins using your recipes in the gluten-free cookbooks! . . . I've never been much of a desserts or sweets fancier, but I sure am now. I love making the different breads in the GF cookbooks as well."

— Larry Ference, Langley, British Columbia

"I love that you use the more nutritious alternative flours, as the old gluten-free standards I find to be very high in carbohydrates and much less nutritious. I have only been on the gluten-free diet for about a year and a half, but I have been a diabetic for almost 29 years."

— Natile Trefan, western Canada

"Donna and Heather's cookbooks are a *must have* for anyone on a gluten-free diet. The recipes are easy to follow, use nutritious gluten-free flours and will be enjoyed by the whole family!"

— Shelley Case, RD, author of *Gluten-Free Diet: A Comprehensive Resource Guide*

Complete
Gluten-Free
Cookbook

Complete
Gluten-Free
Cookbook

150 Gluten-Free, Lactose-Free Recipes, Many with Egg-Free Variations

Donna Washburn & Heather Butt

Robert
ROSE

For complete cataloguing information, see page 304.

Disclaimer
The recipes in this book have been carefully tested. To the best of our knowledge, they are
safe and nutritious for ordinary use and users. All the recipes within this book are gluten-free
according to the Canadian Celiac Association dietary guidelines and based on reasonable
research for accuracy at the time of writing. For those people with food or other allergies, or who
have special food requirements or health issues, please read the suggested contents of each recipe
carefully and determine whether or not they may create a problem for you. All recipes are used
at the risk of the consumer.

We cannot be responsible for any hazards, loss or damage that may occur as a result of any
recipe use.

For those with special needs, allergies, requirements or health problems, in the event of any
doubt, please contact your medical adviser prior to the use of any recipe.

Design & Production: PageWave Graphics Inc.
Editor: Sue Sumeraj
Proofreader: Sheila Wawanash
Recipe Tester: Jennifer MacKenzie
Indexer: Gillian Watts
Photography: Colin Erricson
Food Stylist: Kate Bush
Props Stylist: Charlene Erricson

Cover image: Oatmeal Raisin Cookies (page 268) and Cherry Almond Biscotti (page 274)

We acknowledge the financial support of the Government of Canada through the Book Publishing
Industry Development Program (BPIDP) for our publishing activities.

Published by: Robert Rose Inc.
120 Eglinton Ave. E., Suite 800, Toronto, Ontario, Canada M4P 1E2
Tel: (416) 322-6552   Fax: (416) 322-6936

Printed in Canada
4 5 6 7 8 9 10   TCP   16 15 14 13 12 11 10 09

We dedicate this book to the memory of Carol Coulter.
Carol personified many qualities we admire.
She was a mentor, an inspiration, a loving wife and mother,
a caregiver, a friend and a celiac. We miss her.

Contents

Acknowledgments

This book has had the support and assistance of many people from its inception to the final reality.

Our thanks to the following for supplying products for recipe development: Doug Yuen of Dainty Foods for an assortment of rice, brown rice flour and rice bran; George Birinyi Jr. of Grain Process Enterprises for potato and tapioca starches, xanthan gum, sorghum flour, amaranth flour, bean flour, pea flour and quinoa grain; Chuck Cundari of Canbrands Specialty Foods for Kingsmill Egg Replacer; Raj Sukul of Maple Grove Food & Beverage Corporation for Pastato pasta; Ivan Shih of Rizopia Food Products for a variety of rice pastas; Mai Tucker of National Importers for Want-Want SuperSlim Rice Crisps and Want-Want SuperSlim Brown Rice Crisps; Howard Selig of Valley Flax Flour for flax flour; Margaret Hudson of Burnbrae Farms for Naturegg Simply Egg Whites and Naturegg Break-Free liquid eggs; the employees and owners of *The Baker's Catalogue* of King Arthur Flour for nut flours and dried cranberries; Wendi Hiebert of Ontario Egg Producers for whole-shell eggs; Corey Clack-Streef of Faye Clack Communications for California walnuts and Southern United States Trade Association pecans; Michel Dion of Lallemand for Eagle and Fermipan yeast; Soyaworld for So Nice soy beverage; Beth Armour of Cream Hill Estates for oat flour and oat flakes; Gluten Free Oats for old-fashioned rolled oats; and Andrew Milligan of Hamilton Beach for products for conference draws.

Thank you to the many manufacturers of bread machines who continue to supply the latest models to our test kitchen: Toastmaster, Breadman, Black & Decker, Cuisinart, Sunbeam Oster and Zojirushi.

A huge thank you to the members of our focus group who faithfully and tirelessly tasted and tested gluten-free recipes and products from beginning to end of recipe development. Your comments, suggestions and critical analysis were invaluable and helped make this a better book. Special thanks to Cathy Maggio-Howley and her family, Carol Coulter, Deanna Jennett, Mike of New Horizons, Louella Smail and Leslie Disheau of Lou's Pantry, Madelyn Smith of the Gluten Intolerance Group, Mary Schluckebier of CSA/USA and Shelley Case, RD, for their assistance.

We want to express our appreciation to photographer Colin Erricson, food stylist Kate Bush and prop stylist Charlene Erricson. Thank you for making the photographs of our gluten-free products as delicious-looking as possible. Once again, we enjoyed baking for the photo shoot.

Bob Dees, our publisher, Marian Jarkovich, Sales and Marketing Manager, National Retail Accounts, and Arden Boehm, International Sales and Marketing, at Robert Rose Inc. deserve special thanks for their ongoing support.

To Andrew Smith, Kevin Cockburn and Joseph Gisini of PageWave Graphics, thank you for working through this cookbook's design, layout and production. Thank you to Sue Sumeraj, our editor, and Jennifer MacKenzie, our recipe tester. A very special thanks to Magda Fahmy-Turnbull, RD, for her work on the nutritional analysis. She has been an invaluable resource throughout this project.

Thank you to our families, Heather's husband, our sons, daughters-in-law and grandsons. You helped bring balance to our lives when we became too focused on our work.

And finally, to you, who must follow a gluten-free diet, we sincerely hope these recipes help make your life easier and more enjoyable. We developed them with you in mind.

Introduction

This afternoon at lunch we were sitting outside in the sun, enjoying a GF, LF, EF* Chocolate Chip Muffin — even licking our fingers and wanting seconds. We began reminiscing about the past 20-plus years. Who could have predicted the twists and turns our lives would take?

We first met while team-teaching at a local community college and very quickly formed a strong friendship. Donna pointed out what fun it would be to work together in our own business — not on opposite shifts, but really together. That dream took a few years to realize, however, as Donna continued to teach full-time.

In 1992, Quality Professional Services became a reality, and we spent the next several years developing bread machine recipes for manufacturers and yeast companies and writing bread machine cookbooks. Soon enough, emails, phone calls and letters poured in from celiacs wanting GF bread recipes. Accepting the challenge was a major commitment, shifting us right out of our comfort zone, but we jumped in with both feet.

Today, as we work and travel to conferences together, our friendship continues to grow stronger. We laugh when we are tired, and finish each other's sentences. We both love to eat and hate to file.

One of our dearest celiac friends, Carol Coulter, passed away this year. Heather met Carol while eating fish and chips in Whitehorse, Yukon, when we were researching our first gluten-free cookbook. An immediate friend, Carol was a font of information and knowledge, which she willingly shared. Over the years, we learned that Carol helped many celiacs in the London, Ontario, area with recipes, advice and encouragement. For each of our cookbooks, Carol shared a recipe with us, which we adapted for you: in *125 Best Gluten-Free Recipes* it was the Batter-Fried Fish; in *The Best Gluten-Free Family Cookbook* it was Carol's Fruit Cake; and for this one it's a not-so-low-calorie brownie (Carol's Brownies, page 276). Her husband, Gary, and daughter, Pam, say, "After being diagnosed with celiac disease, she was truly a champion of the cause. In true Mom spirit, she would spend hours talking to newly diagnosed celiacs, sharing recipes, giving samples away and just being a friend they could call when recipes didn't turn out, or they needed advice on how to eat in restaurants, or they just needed to chat." We dedicated this book to Carol because she personified what it means to be a friend and a celiac.

One of the best perks of working on a gluten-free cookbook is that we get to meet and talk with you, our readers. You challenge us with your requests, inspire us with your commitment and reinvigorate us with your enthusiasm. For *Complete Gluten-Free Cookbook*, we listened when you asked for recipes that were lactose-free and egg-free, and we've given you a nutritional analysis for each recipe. We've fulfilled your requests for sourdough breads, donuts, sticky buns you can roll out, and brown dinner rolls, and we've provided muffin recipes that make only a half-dozen. We always personally bake and deliver the food to Toronto for the photographer; that way, you know exactly what to expect from our recipes. We were so pleased with ourselves when we had most of our recipes developed before the hot, hazy, humid days of summer, only to find that, to have food ready for the photos, we had to bake from early morning to late at night on a day of record-breaking heat and humidity!

As we develop recipes and research new flours and grains, we realize the importance of lifelong learning and accepting new challenges — it keeps us fresh and young!

Please keep in touch with us.

Donna J. Washburn, P.H.Ec., and Heather L. Butt, P.H.Ec.
Quality Professional Services
1104 Burnside Drive
Brockville, Ontario K6V 5T1

Phone/fax: (613) 923-2116
Email: bread@ripnet.com
Website: www.bestbreadrecipes.com

* gluten-free, lactose-free, egg-free

Speaking Our Language: Are We All on the Same Page?

1. "GF" means "gluten-free," such as GF sour cream, GF mayonnaise, etc., when both gluten-free and gluten-containing products are available. We recommend that you read package labels every time you purchase a GF product. Manufacturers frequently change the formulas and ingredients of prepared products.

♦

2. Our recipes were developed with both lactose-free and lactose-containing products: lactose-free milk, soy beverage and regular cow's milk (we tested with 2%, 1% or nonfat, but our recipes will work with other levels of fat); buttery spread and salted butter; soy yogurt and yogurt; and sour cream and cream cheese substitutes as well as sour cream and cream cheese.

♦

3. In developing our recipes, we used large eggs, liquid honey, fancy (not blackstrap) molasses, bread machine (instant) yeast and unsweetened fruit juice (not fruit drinks). We know you'll get the same great results if you bake with these; expect slightly different results if you make substitutions.

♦

4. Unless otherwise stated in the recipe, eggs, lactose-free products and regular dairy products are used cold from the refrigerator.

♦

5. If the preparation method (chop, melt, dice, slice, etc.) is listed before the food, it means you prepare the food before measuring. If it is listed after the food, measure first, then prepare. Examples are "ground flaxseed" vs. "flaxseed, ground" and "cooked brown rice" vs. "brown rice, cooked."

6. Select either metric or imperial measures and stick to one for the whole recipe; do not mix.

♦

7. Use measuring spoons for small amounts. New sets on the market include smidgeon, pinch, dash, $\frac{1}{8}$ tsp, $\frac{1}{2}$ tbsp, 2 tsp and 2 tbsp, in addition to the traditional $\frac{1}{4}$ tsp, $\frac{1}{2}$ tsp, 1 tsp and 1 tbsp. The metric small measures are available in 1 mL, 2 mL, 5 mL, 15 mL and 25 mL sizes. There are also sets of long-handled, narrow spoons made especially to fit into spice jars. These are accurate and fun to use.

♦

8. We use the "spoon lightly into the correct dry measuring cup (the nesting style), heap the top and level once" method of measuring for accuracy and perfect products. Do not pack or tap the cup before leveling.

♦

9. Use a graduated, clear liquid measuring cup (with a spout and handle) for all liquids. Place on a flat surface and read at eye level.

♦

10. If in doubt about a food term, a piece of equipment or a specific recipe technique, refer to the glossaries located on pages 291 to 302.

♦

11. All foods that require washing are washed before preparation. Foods such as onions, garlic and bananas are peeled, but fresh peaches and apples are not, unless specified.

Understanding Whole Grains

"A whole grain is the entire seed, including the naturally occurring nutrients of an edible plant. The size, shape and color of the seed, also referred to as the 'kernel,' varies with the species. A grain is considered a whole grain when it contains all three primary seed parts: bran, germ and endosperm."

— The Whole Grains Council

What Is Meant by "Whole Grain"?

As the quote above explains, a whole grain consists of three parts: the bran, the germ and the endosperm. The **bran**, or outer coating, is made up of several layers. It encloses the seed to protect it from moisture, pests, disease, light and air. It is rich in insoluble fiber and contains antioxidants and B vitamins. Just beneath the bran layers is a small structure called the **germ**. This is the part of the seed that grows into a new plant. The germ is rich in healthy oils, B vitamins, minerals including magnesium and iron, and some protein. The main component of the grain, the **endosperm**, is also the largest part. It contains starch, protein, soluble fiber and small amounts of vitamins and minerals.

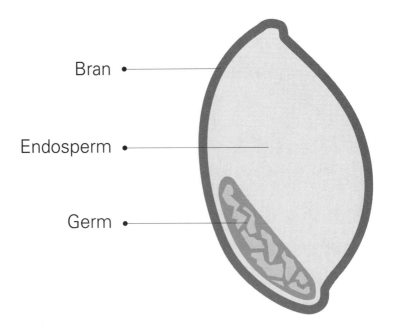

Bran

Endosperm

Germ

Whole grains contain all three parts, whereas refined grains (white rice, defatted soy, degerminated cornmeal) have the bran and germ removed, leaving only the endosperm, although they keep their seed-like shape. Refined grains are thus nutritionally inferior to whole grains. Some refined grains may be enriched (some of the nutrients that were removed are added back), but not all GF grains, flours or products such as cereals and pasta are enriched. It is very important to read labels when purchasing products made commercially with GF flours.

Whole grains can be eaten whole, cracked, ground or milled into flour. They can be the basis of commercial pastas, cereals and baked products. A whole grain that has been processed (cracked, crushed, ground, milled, rolled, extruded and/or cooked) should deliver approximately the same rich balance of nutrients found in the original grain seed.

Flour is the ground form of a grain. It can be milled from the whole grain or may be a refined and processed grain. Look for a label that states "100% whole grain," not just "whole grain" — the latter may contain only a small proportion of whole grains.

Can Celiacs Eat Whole Grains?

Gluten-intolerant people *can* eat whole grains. A large number of GF whole-grain choices are available. The following, when eaten in a form that includes the bran, germ and endosperm, are examples of generally accepted GF whole-grain foods:

- amaranth
- buckwheat
- corn, including whole cornmeal
- millet
- Montina (Indian rice grass)
- oats, including oatmeal
- quinoa
- rice, both brown and colored, and wild rice
- sorghum
- teff

(Approved and endorsed by the Whole Grains Council, May 2004, www.wholegrainscouncil.org)

How Much Should I Eat?

The U.S. Department of Agriculture's MyPyramid recommends that adults eat a total of 6 ounces (175 g) of grains a day (based on a 2,000-calorie diet). At least 3 ounces (90 g) of this should include whole-grain cereals, breads, crackers, rice or pasta. One ounce (30 g) equals 1 slice of bread, 1 cup (250 mL) of breakfast cereal or ½ cup (125 mL) of cooked rice, cereal or pasta (**www.mypyramid.gov**).

Canada's Food Guide to Healthy Eating (presently under revision) recommends that adults eat 5 to 12 servings from the grain products group each day. Of these, health experts suggest that at least 3 servings be whole-grain products. One serving is 1 slice of bread, 1 ounce (30 g) of cold cereal, ¾ cup (175 mL) of hot cereal or ½ cup (125 mL) of pasta or rice (**www.hc-sc.gc.ca/fn-an/food-guide-aliment/index_e.html**).

How Can I Combine Grains with Other Foods to Create a Complete Protein?

Meat, fish and poultry, milk and milk products and eggs are considered complete proteins, as they contain all of the essential amino acids necessary for a healthy body. The type of protein found in grains is considered incomplete, as it does not contain all the essential amino acids needed. However, the body has the ability to use amino acids from a variety of sources to form complete proteins. Here are some suggested combinations: beans and rice, cereals and milk, nuts and grains, and/or whole-grain breads and legumes.

All grains are not created equal: some contain more and higher levels of essential amino acids than others. Check the "Nutritional Value" section of each of the gluten-free grains in "The Gluten-Free Pantry" (pages 19–61) for more specific information on the amino acids and other important nutrients the grains provide.

The Gluten-Free Pantry

We developed the recipes in this book using the gluten-free grains, as well as nutritious nuts, beans, seeds, flax and soy. Some of these ingredients are used whole to make deliciously healthy salads and side dishes, while others are ground into flour for flavorful baked goods such as pizza crusts, breads and desserts. In this section, you'll find all the information you need on each of these ingredients, from notes on their history and details on their appearance, flavor and texture to suggestions on how to use them and instructions on how to store them. We also tell you their nutritional value and list some websites where you can go to learn more.

Amaranth

Amaranth, an 8,000-year-old crop, was called the "super food" by the Aztecs, who believed it made them invincible. It was a staple of their culture until Cortés decreed that anyone growing it would be put to death. However, seeds were smuggled to Asia, where amaranth became known in local dialects as "king seed" and "seed sent by God" as a tribute to its taste and sustenance. Twenty years ago, the "ancient crop with a future" enjoyed a renaissance when the National Academy of Sciences recommended amaranth as one of 20 foods to be reintroduced into the American diet. Currently, amaranth is grown in Mexico, Peru and Nepal, as well as in the United States.

Not a true cereal grain, amaranth is sometimes called a "pseudo-grain." It is closely related to the goosefoot family, which also includes pigweed, spinach and beets.

Forms of Amaranth

- **Amaranth seeds** (also known as whole-grain amaranth) are off-white, golden, tan or light brown in color and are about the size of poppy seeds. The flavor ranges from mild, slightly sweet, nutty, toasty and malt-like to a more robust, peppery whole-grain taste.
- **Amaranth flour** is very fine and has a light cream color and a pleasant, nutty, toasted taste. Because of its high moisture content, it is best mixed with other flours. It produces goods that are moist and dense, but the use of starch helps

lighten the texture. The grain of the bread is more open, the texture not as silky and the crumb color slightly darker than wheat flour breads. Amaranth flour tends to form a crust on the outside of a product during baking, sealing the outside before the product is completely cooked on the inside, so use the smallest amount of liquid you can and allow for slightly longer baking times than you might otherwise. Products baked with amaranth tend to brown quickly and may need to be tented during the last third of the baking time.

- **Toasted amaranth bran flour** has a mild, nutty flavor. It can replace amaranth flour cup for cup (mL for mL) in baking.

Use

- Amaranth seeds are extremely versatile in recipes for breads, pastries and other baked goods. Raw seeds can be left whole or ground.
- To make a breakfast cereal or a side dish, combine 1 part amaranth seeds with 2 parts water or GF stock; simmer gently for 20 minutes. Stir almost constantly or lumps will form. Cooked amaranth has a sticky texture as compared to cooked rice and other grains. Be careful not to overcook it, as it becomes very gummy.
- Stews and soups can be thickened by adding a small amount of amaranth seeds.
- Use amaranth seeds in crackers, granola, breading, crusts, toppings for casseroles and confections with molasses or honey.
- Amaranth flour makes great-tasting bread, muffins, cookies, pancakes, flatbreads and donuts. The flavor complements nut flours.
- Amaranth flour is one of our favorites for thickening gravy, as it results in a dull finish and holds well (see "Thickener Substitutions," page 57).

Storage

Store amaranth seeds in an airtight container in a cool, dry, dark place for up to 1 month, refrigerate for up to 6 months or freeze for up to 1 year. Cooked amaranth seeds can be stored, covered, in the refrigerator, but should be used within a few days or frozen for up to 6 months. Refrigerate amaranth flour for up to 6 months or freeze for up to 1 year.

Nutritional Value

Like all other whole grains, amaranth supplies protein, carbohydrate, dietary fiber, B vitamins (thiamine, riboflavin niacin, folate) and minerals (iron, zinc and magnesium). It also contributes calcium, phosphorus and potassium. Amaranth contains lysine, an amino acid missing in many grains, giving it a high level of protein. In addition to its outstanding nutritional value, it is very low in sodium and contains no saturated fat. The grain contains more fiber and iron than wheat.

Further Information

- www.innvista.com
- www.msnbc.com
- www.nuworldamaranth.com
- www.specialfoods.com
- www.waltonfeed.com

Buckwheat

Buckwheat (also known as saracen corn) is thought to have originated in China or Central Asia, where it still grows wild today. It is widely grown in Canada and the Soviet Union, but is a relatively minor crop in the United States. For centuries, buckwheat was a major food source for Japanese people living in mountainous regions, where the climate and soil weren't good for growing rice.

Buckwheat is not officially a grain, a grass or a wheat, but is related to rhubarb and sorrel. The three-cornered (triangular) seed kernels are covered with a black shell.

Forms of Buckwheat

- **Buckwheat groats** are the hulled, mild-flavored, soft, white seeds (kernels) of the buckwheat plant. They are available whole or cracked into coarse, medium or fine grinds. Finely cracked groats are called **grits**, which may be labeled "cream of buckwheat."
- **Kasha** is made by roasting or toasting buckwheat groats. The groats become darker in color and the nutty flavor becomes stronger.
- **Buckwheat flakes** (oatmeal-style) are rolled flakes made from buckwheat groats treated with hot steam. These small, brittle flakes have the appearance of small rolled oats with a slightly sweeter flavor and a slightly browner color.

- **Buckwheat flour** is made by finely grinding groats. You can make your own by processing groats in a blender or food processor to a fine powder. It has a unique, strong, musty, slightly sour, slightly nutty flavor. Light buckwheat flour has the hull removed before milling. Dark buckwheat flour, ground from unhulled seeds, is grayish with tiny black specks and has a stronger taste due to the presence of the finely milled hull particles. Buckwheat flour tends to make baked goods heavier and give them a distinctive, stronger taste. It is most often blended with other flours.

> Buckwheat blossoms, rich in nectar, make an excellent honey. Some beekeepers plant buckwheat just for the honey.

Use

- Groats can be cooked quickly and served as you would rice, or can be combined with rice to dilute their intense flavor. To cook, thoroughly rinse 1/2 cup (125 mL) groats, then combine with 1 cup (250 mL) water and simmer for 15 to 20 minutes, or until groats have tripled in volume.
- In Eastern Europe, and especially in Russia, buckwheat groats are made into a nutritious porridge, served hot for breakfast.
- Kasha is used in dishes ranging from pilafs to meat mixtures.
- Buckwheat flakes can be added as you would rolled oats to any GF recipe, or served as a porridge or muesli.
- Buckwheat flour is used in pancake mixes, Russian blinis, Japanese soba noodles (which contain wheat), crêpes, dumplings, unleavened chapatis and pastries. It can be used as a meat extender in a sausage meat mixture or combined with other GF flours to make breads and quick breads.

> Some people have difficulty digesting buckwheat.

Storage

Store buckwheat flakes in an airtight container in a cool, dry place for up to 2 years. Refrigerate groats, grits, kasha and buckwheat flour for up to 6 months or freeze for up to 1 year.

Nutritional Value

Like all other whole grains, buckwheat supplies protein, carbohydrate, dietary fiber, B vitamins (thiamine, niacin, riboflavin and folate) and minerals (iron, zinc and magnesium). It also contributes phosphorous, vitamin B_6 and potassium. Like amaranth, buckwheat is a source of lysine, an amino acid commonly lacking in the true cereal grains. In addition, it surpasses corn in all of the essential amino acids and supplies more calcium and vitamin B_6 than wheat.

Further Information
- www.innvista.com
- www.recipetips.com
- www.theglutenfreelifestyle.com

Corn

For thousands of years, the Hopi and the Navajo made blue cornmeal from a variety of blue-black corn. Traditionally, it has been said that those living north of the Mason-Dixon Line eat yellow cornmeal, and those living south of it eat white cornmeal and feed the yellow corn to the hogs!

Forms of Corn
- **Cornmeal** (polenta) is a flour-like substance milled from corn. It has larger granules than regular flour and can be yellow (the most common), white, blue or red. The grind may be fine, medium or coarse. The coarser the grind, the more granular the texture of the finished product and the more intense the corn flavor. Check labels of commercial products for the addition of wheat.
- **White cornmeal** is ground from whole-grain white corn to a medium coarseness. Although a little more delicate in flavor, it can replace yellow in any baked product.
- **Yellow cornmeal** is a bit sweeter and "cornier" in flavor than white cornmeal. It is traditionally used for cornbread.
- **Blue cornmeal**, a dark indigo blue, is a bit coarser than yellow or white meal, and has a somewhat sweeter, more intense corn flavor. It is used to make purple pancakes, muffins and cornbread and can be substituted for yellow in any recipe.
- **Stone-ground cornmeal** is produced by crushing corn kernels under a millstone, retaining the germ. Fresh stone-ground cornmeal has a rich corn flavor.
- **Degerminated cornmeal** is ground between massive steel rollers. The fiber and corn germ are separated out, leaving a less nutritious and less flavorful grain. Avoid products that are labeled "degerminated" when you're looking for whole-grain cornmeal.

Corn flour and cornstarch are not interchangeable in recipes.

Because cornmeal swells during cooking, 1 cup (250 mL) of dry cornmeal makes about 4 cups (1 L) of cooked cornmeal.

- **Corn flour** contains the whole grain — bran, germ and endosperm — and is more finely ground than cornmeal. Atole flour, harinilla and masa harina are among the different types of corn flour commonly produced. The variety of corn used and the degree to which it is milled and processed determine the type of flour. Degerminated corn flour is also available.

Use

- Cornmeal can be used to make cornbread, spoon bread, corn sticks and muffins, or cooked and served as a hot cereal or side dish (polenta). It also can be used as a coating for fried foods or as a meat extender.
- Baked goods made using corn flour have a lighter texture than those made with the coarser cornmeal. Cornbread made with corn flour is richer and less crumbly.

Storage

Store cornmeal and corn flour in airtight containers in a cool, dry, dark place for up to 1 month, refrigerate for up to 6 months or freeze for up to 1 year. Degerminated cornmeal and corn flour have a longer shelf life because the germ, including the oil, has been removed; they can be stored at room temperature for up to 6 months.

Nutritional Value

Like all other whole grains, cornmeal and corn flour supply protein, carbohydrate, dietary fiber, B vitamins (thiamine, riboflavin, niacin, folate) and minerals (iron, manganese, phosphorus and magnesium). However, different colors provide different amounts, with blue being highest in protein, iron, manganese and phosphorus. A new study shows that corn has the highest level of antioxidants of any grain or vegetable — almost twice the antioxidant activity of apples!

Degerminated cornmeal and corn flour are enriched with iron and three B vitamins. Some cornmeal is enriched with calcium and vitamin D.

Further Information

- www.muextension.missouri.edu
- www.wareaglemill.com

Flaxseed

Flax is one of the oldest cultivated crops. Ten thousand years ago, Swiss lake dwellers extracted fiber from flax stalks to use for clothing, ropes and nets. Flax was first brought to North America in 1617. Grown on the prairies in Canada and the north-central United States, it produces soft, blue flowers.

Forms of Flaxseed

- **Whole flaxseed** (also known as linseed) refers to the unbroken seed. The seeds are small, flat and tear-shaped. They range in color from dark reddish-brown to golden and have a nutty flavor and a crisp, yet chewy texture. Flaxseed should be shiny and very oily on the surface.
- **Cracked flaxseed** is not sold in stores but can be created at home: use a coffee grinder to crack the outer coating of the seed slightly, resulting in pieces of different sizes and textures. Cracked flaxseed is easier to digest than whole flaxseed.
- **Ground flaxseed** is sold as flax flour, milled flaxseed or sprouted flax flour. You can also make your own by grinding whole flaxseed to a medium brown powder with slightly darker flecks. All forms of ground flaxseed are interchangeable in recipes.

Use a coffee grinder or food processor to crack or grind whole flaxseed to the consistency you want for your recipe. For optimum freshness, it is best to grind it as you need it.

Use

- Add whole flaxseed to yeast breads and quick breads or sprinkle on salads and cereals (both hot and cold).
- Crack whole flaxseed slightly to add crunch to a bread or muffin, or grind to the consistency of coarsely ground coffee for use in muffins, breads or cakes.
- Sprinkle cracked flaxseed on cereal, salad, ice cream or puddings. Add just before serving, as it becomes sticky.
- Ground flaxseed acts as a tenderizer for yeast breads.
- Replace up to 1/3 cup (75 mL) of vegetable oil in recipes with 1 cup (250 mL) of flax flour or ground flaxseed.
- You can add up to 1 tbsp (15 mL) flax flour or ground flaxseed to any baked product (such as cookies, cakes and pancakes) without decreasing the other flour. If you add more, the amount of liquid and other flours may have to be adjusted.

See "Egg-Free Baking," page 65, for instructions on substituting ground flaxseed for eggs.

Storage

Whole flaxseed can be stored at room temperature for up to 1 year. Store cracked flaxseed, ground flaxseed and flax flour in the refrigerator for up to 6 months.

Nutritional Value

Flaxseed contains protein, polyunsaturated fat, soluble and insoluble fiber and lignans. It is rich in omega-3 fatty acids, B vitamins, and minerals including iron, calcium, magnesium, phosphorus, copper, zinc, potassium and manganese. Brown and gold seeds are nutritionally equal. The seeds need to be cracked or ground for the body to use the nutrients efficiently.

Further Information

- www.flaxcouncil.ca
- www.flaxflour.com
- www.saskflax.com

Hemp Seed

Hemp (*Cannabis sativa*) has been cultivated for centuries as fiber for rope, sails and clothing. Today, the seed is crushed to provide a source of oil, food and animal feed.

Forms of Hemp Seed

- **Hulled hemp seeds** (hemp seed nuts, Hemp Hearts, hemp nuts) are the whole seeds with the crunchy outer shell removed. Raw organic hulled whole hemp seeds are often called hemp protein or hulled hemp protein. They are deep green and have a pleasant, nutty flavor similar to that of sunflower seeds.
- **Hemp seed flour** is sometimes called hemp protein powder, powdered hemp protein or hemp pro. Its natural nuttiness adds a pleasant flavor to any drink you whip up.

Use

- Hulled hemp seeds can be sprinkled on top of hot or cold cereal, stir-fries or ice cream. They can be blended into sandwich fillings, spreads or dips for a nutty flavor, or baked into cookies, breads and pastries for added crunch (however, the fat may have to be reduced because of the high fat content of the seeds).

- Hemp seed flour can be used to make pancakes, cookies, muffins, brownies or breads. For best results, it should be blended with other flours.

Hulled hemp seeds and flaxseed are interchangeable in recipes.

Storage

Purchase hulled hemp seeds and hemp seed flour only from stores that sell refrigerated products. Keep refrigerated once open and use within 1 year.

Nutritional Value

Hemp seed is high in protein, polyunsaturated fat, omega-3 and omega-6 fatty acids, dietary fiber and iron.

Further Information

- www.hempseed.ca
- www.hempola.com
- www.manitobaharvest.com
- www.rawganique.com

Legumes

The history of legumes (peas, beans, lentils and peanuts) spans the globe. Some archaeologists think that people started growing peas and lentils more than 20,000 years ago. Peas have been found in caves in Thailand that are over 11,000 years old. Lentils are a staple in Middle Eastern and Indian cooking. Christopher Columbus is believed to have brought the first peas to America in 1493, planting them on Isabella Island. French settlers brought hearty pea soup with them when they arrived in North America, and baked beans were considered a staple for western ranchers riding the winter trail.

Legumes have pods that split on both sides when ripe. They can be purchased dried, canned, fresh or frozen, but we have used only dried and canned varieties in our recipes. If you can't find a particular dried or canned legume in the store, you can easily substitute another. For example, pinto and black beans are good substitutes for red kidney beans, and cannellini, lima beans and navy beans are interchangeable.

Soybeans are also legumes, but because they have unique qualities, we've dealt with them separately (see page 52).

Types of Dried Legumes

- **Dried beans** are allowed to dry in the pod. There are over 25 different types of dried beans, including pinto beans, kidney beans, black beans, white beans, navy beans and lima beans. Some legumes with the word "pea" in their name, such as chickpeas (garbanzo beans) and black-eyed peas, are actually more closely related to beans than to peas.

- **Dried peas** (split peas or field peas) are allowed to dry naturally in the field before they are harvested. This category of pea includes green peas and yellow peas.
- **Lentils** are the lens-shaped (flattened) seeds of an annual herb, dried as soon as they're ripe. They are sold with and without husks and come in many different colors, including brown, red and green.

Use

- Once they've been soaked and cooked (see below), versatile dried legumes can be served as a side dish, puréed or processed into oils or butters. Because they are high in protein, they are often used as a meat substitute in soups, stews and casseroles.
- Lentils make a quick substitute for meat in spaghetti sauce and are an integral part of East Indian dal.
- Lentil and pea purées have a similar texture to pumpkin purée and can be used in baked goods to increase the nutritional value.
- Puréed beans make an excellent base for dips and spreads. Hummus, made from puréed chickpeas, can be used as a sandwich filling or a dip for veggies, or can be added hot to soups and side dishes.

Soaking Dried Legumes

Except for lentils, mung beans and split peas, all dried legumes need to be soaked before they can be cooked. Soaking rehydrates them for more even cooking and reduces the indigestible complex sugar that causes gas (flatulence).

First, sort and rinse dried beans or whole peas, then combine them with water. A general rule of thumb is to use 3 cups (750 mL) of water for each 1 cup (250 mL) of dried beans or whole peas. Select one of the following three soaking methods:

- **Overnight Soak:** Choose this traditional method when you have more time. The beans will hold their shape better, have a more uniform texture and need less cooking time. Place water and beans in a large casserole dish, cover and let stand on the counter overnight.

- **Quick Soak:** Choose this method when you need to cook beans the same day. Place water and beans in a large saucepan, bring to a full boil and boil for 2 minutes. Remove from heat, cover and let stand for 2 hours.
- **Microwave Soak:** Choose this method to cut the Quick Soak time in half. Place water and beans in a large microwave-safe casserole dish and microwave on High for 10 to 15 minutes, or until boiling. Cover and let stand for 1 hour.

To reduce the gas-producing properties of beans, always discard the soaking liquid and cook the beans in fresh water.

Cooking Legumes

Soaked legumes can be cooked on the stovetop, in the microwave or in a slow cooker or pressure cooker. Again, use 3 cups (750 mL) of water for each 1 cup (250 mL) of dried beans or whole peas. Here are some tips:

Beans more than double in size after soaking and cooking.

- Simmer beans gently — boiling tends to split the skins.
- To reduce foaming and boiling over, add 1 tbsp (15 mL) of buttery spread, butter, margarine or oil to the cooking water.
- Cook legumes until al dente — soft enough to eat but not overdone.
- If you are cooking legumes in aluminum or cast iron pans, using hard water or cooking at high altitudes, you will need to increase both soaking and cooking times.
- If your pot is not covered, you will need to stir the legumes occasionally, and you may need to add more water partway through.
- To cut down on the earthy flavor of dried beans and peas, add freshly squeezed lemon juice at the end of the cooking time and/or cook in meat or vegetable stock.
- To preserve the color of split peas, add a small amount of fresh gingerroot to the cooking water.

Because canned beans are already cooked, they only need reheating for about a minute.

- When cooking bean dishes, add salty, acidic and dairy ingredients at the end of the cooking time. Acids (such as tomatoes, lemon juice and vinegar), salt and calcium react with the bean surface, preventing water from entering the bean and cooking the starch.

1 lb (500 g) dried beans = about 2 cups (500 mL) = 4 to 6 cups (1 to 1.5 L) cooked

1 lb (500 g) dried split peas = about 2⅓ cups (575 mL) = about 5 cups (1.25 L) cooked

1 lb (500 g) dried lentils = about 2¼ cups (550 mL) = 3 to 3½ cups (750 to 875 mL) cooked

Storage

Store dried legumes in a dry, airtight container at room temperature for up to 1 year. Beans lose moisture over time and take longer to soak and cook. Do not store dried beans in the refrigerator.

Store unopened canned legumes in a cool, dry place for up to 5 years.

Refrigerate cooked beans for up to 5 days or freeze for up to 6 months. Refrigerate cooked lentils or split peas for up to 4 days or freeze for up to 6 months. Defrost beans, lentils and peas in the refrigerator.

Nutritional Value

Legumes are a source of protein, complex carbohydrate, calcium, iron, B vitamins (especially folate) and both soluble and insoluble fiber. Romano beans have the highest folate count of all beans.

Further Information

- http://beprepared.com
- www.celiacpeterborough.ca
- www.farmbuilt.com
- www.ocbga.com

Legume Flours

Legume flours been recently been introduced to celiacs for use in GF baking, expanding your choices and increasing the nutrition of baked goods. To make these flours, dried peas and beans are heat-treated to help reduce flatulence, then ground into flour. (For information on soy flour, see page 52.)

Types of Legume Flours

- **Fava bean flour** is a fine-textured flour made from earthy-flavored fava beans (sometimes confused with lima beans). Before milling, the beans are blanched to remove their tough, wrinkled, dark brown skins.
- **Chickpea flour** (garbanzo bean flour, gram, besan, chana) adds a rich, sweet flavor to baked foods. It is brownish yellow and has a mild, nut-like taste, with a hint of lemon.
- **Garfava flour** (sold as garbanzo-fava bean flour in Canada) is a blend of garbanzo bean (chickpea) flour and fava bean flour. It has a light tan color and a nutty taste.

- **Whole bean flour** is made from Romano beans (also called cranberry beans or speckled sugar beans). The dried beans are cooked (micronized), then stone-ground to a uniform, fine, dark, strong-tasting flour, with nothing wasted in the milling process. When one of our recipes calls for whole bean flour, use this one; however, if it's not available, any bean or pea flour can be substituted.
- **White (navy) bean flour** is made from small, white round or oval beans. The white flour has a mild flavor and a powdery texture.
- **Pinto bean flour** has a slightly pink tinge, although the pinto beans it is made from have a spotty beige and brown color.
- **Pea flours** are produced from selected dried field peas with the bran (hull) removed. The flours are silky soft and the color of the pea they are made from. Green pea flour has a sweeter flavor than yellow pea flour.

> All types of bean flours (except soy flour) can be used interchangeably with pea flours in our recipes.

Use

- Legume flours combine well with other GF flours. They complement recipes made with molasses, brown sugar, chocolate, pumpkin and applesauce.
- Chickpea flour is most often used in East Indian cuisine. It can be substituted for soy flour in most recipes.
- Yellow and green pea flours keep baked products softer longer, improve dough made in a bread machine and reduce mixing times.
- Pea flours can be used as a natural colorant in baked goods, homemade noodles and other foods. They complement recipes made with banana, peanut butter and strong spices such as cloves.

Storage
Refrigerate legume flours for up to 6 months or freeze for up to 1 year.

Nutritional Value
Bean and pea flours offer the same nutritional benefits as the bean or pea they are made from. All are a source of protein. Whole bean flour provides more calcium, iron, potassium, thiamine, riboflavin, folate, fat and dietary fiber than all-purpose wheat flour or any other GF flour except for soybean flour.

Further Information
- http://beprepared.com
- www.celiacpeterborough.ca
- www.farmbuilt.com
- www.foodprocessing.com

Millet

Millet is one of the oldest foods, and possibly the first cereal grain, dating back to 5500 BC in China. It has been a staple in Africa and India for thousands of years. Today, millet ranks as the sixth most important grain in the world, giving sustenance to a third of the world's population.

A member of the Gramineae family, millet is not a true grain but is closely related to corn and sorghum. There are many varieties of millet, but the four major types are pearl, foxtail, proso and finger. Pearl millet produces the largest seeds and is the variety most commonly used for human consumption. It is available as a whole grain, grits, a meal and a flour. Because of its hard, indigestible hull, millet must be hulled before it can be eaten. Hulling does not affect the nutrient value, as the germ stays intact through this process.

Yellow pearl millet, the most common in North America, has a sweet, light, delicate, corn-like flavor. The small, round seeds are about ¾ inch (2 cm) in diameter. They can be gray, red, yellow or white. Once out of the hull, the grains look like tiny yellow spheres with a dot on one side where they were attached to the stem.

Forms of Millet

Steam whole millet grain in a steamer for best results. The grain has a fluffier texture when less water is used; otherwise, it can be very moist and dense.

- **Millet grain** has a mild flavor and a texture much like brown rice. Millet takes on the flavor of whatever it is cooked with.
- **Millet grits** are coarsely ground millet grain. They have a slightly sweet flavor, similar to corn.
- **Millet meal** is more finely ground than millet grits, but more coarsely ground than millet flour.
- **Millet flour** is made from finely ground millet grain. It can be substituted for rice flour in most recipes and adds a lovely cream color to baked goods. A small amount can be substituted for other GF flours, but results may vary.

Use

- Millet grain can be used in pilafs and casseroles, as a stuffing for vegetables and meat, or in Asian dishes that call for rice, quinoa or buckwheat.
- Add millet grain dry to yeast breads, biscuits and muffins for a hint of sweetness and a crunchy texture.
- A small amount of millet grain can be used to thicken and add body to soups and stews.
- Millet grits and millet meal can be added to breads and muffins or sprinkled on salads.
- Millet flour is used in flatbreads or mixed with other flours for baking. It produces light, dry, delicate breads with a thin, buttery smooth crust.

Storage

Refrigerate millet grain, grits, meal and flour for up to 6 months or freeze for up to 1 year.

Nutritional Value

Millet is rich in B vitamins, phosphorus, magnesium, iron, zinc, copper and manganese. Its protein content is a little lower than that of wheat. Like wheat, millet is low in lysine. It is a source of fiber.

Further Information

- www.aaoobfoods.com
- www.chetday.com

Montina

Montina is the registered trade name for flour milled from the seed of a native North American grass called Indian ricegrass (it is not related to rice, despite its name). Native Americans prepared flatbread from the ground seeds. In 2001, the Amazing Grains Grower Cooperative of Montana was formed to grow and market Montina.

Forms of Montina

- **Montina Pure Baking Supplement** is 100% Indian ricegrass, and is used in addition to other GF flours. It is a light brown-gray and is slightly sweet.
- **Montina All-Purpose Flour Blend** is a combination of white rice flour, tapioca flour and Montina Pure.

Use

- Substitute Montina Pure Baking Supplement for 15% to 20% of any other GF flour in a recipe.
- Montina All-Purpose Flour Blend can be used cup for cup (mL for mL) to replace any GF flour or wheat flour. It doesn't need to be mixed with any other GF flour, but xanthan gum must be added. It can be used to make muffins, breads and pancakes and to thicken gravies, soups and stews.

Storage

Montina products can be stored in a cool, dry place for up to 2 years with no deterioration in quality.

Nutritional Value

No complete nutritional analysis has been done to date. Montina Pure Baking Supplement is high in protein, fiber, calcium and iron; however, Montina All-Purpose Flour Blend is much lower in these nutrients.

Further Information

- www.amazinggrains.com

Nuts

Most nuts are the edible seeds or dried fruits of trees; the majority have hard, woody outer husks that protect the softer kernels inside. Walnuts and peanuts are not "true" nuts. Purchase nuts in small amounts, wait until you're ready to use them before you shell or chop them, and always taste them before using. If they're slightly stale, freshen by lightly toasting in the oven.

Types of Nuts

- **Almonds** are referred to several times in the Old Testament and were considered a prize ingredient in the breads served to the Egyptian Pharaohs. Almond trees are believed to have first been cultivated in China and were then brought via the Silk Road to the Middle East and Europe. In the mid-1700s, Franciscan monks planted the first almond trees at California missions. Today, almost all of the almonds grown in the United States are grown in California. Almonds are an ivory-colored nut with a pointed, oval shape and a smooth texture. They have a thin, medium-brown skin that adheres to the nut.

Whole almonds come in both sweet and bitter forms. Sweet almonds are what most bakers are familiar with. They have a delicate taste that is delicious in breads, cookies, cakes, fillings and candies. Almonds are sold either blanched (skins off) or natural (skins on); blanched and natural almonds are interchangeable in recipes. They are also available sliced, slivered or ground. Two cups (500 mL) of almonds weigh about 12 oz (375 g).

See the Technique Glossary, page 299, to learn how to blanch whole almonds.

- **Hazelnuts** have been around for more than 4,500 years. Today, hazelnuts are harvested in Oregon and Washington, though the cultivated variety sometimes known as filberts grows primarily in Turkey, Italy and Spain. The hazelnut has also been known as the cobnut, the Spanish nut, the Pontiac nut and the Lombard. In general, hazelnuts are slightly larger than filberts, and have a weaker flavor. Both nuts have a round, smooth shell and look like small, smooth brown marbles. They are interchangeable in recipes.

For instructions on removing the bitter skin of hazelnuts, see the Technique Glossary, page 300.

- The **pecan** is the only major nut tree indigenous to the United States, dating as far back as the 1500s, when pecans were a major food source for Native Americans. Today, the pecan is one of the most valuable North American nuts. Years of cultivation have produced hundreds of varieties of pecans — small and large, hard-shelled and soft-shelled. The sweet, mellow nut is smooth but ridged, oval, golden brown on the outside and tan on the inside. You can purchase pecans whole, halved, chopped or in chips.

The name "pecan" comes from an Algonquian word meaning "nut requiring a stone to crack."

- **Pine nuts** (*piñons*) were praised as aphrodisiacs by the ancient Greeks and Romans. In North America, pine nuts were a staple in the diets of the Hopi and the Navajo. The small, soft nut is shaped like a teardrop and has a light, delicate, slightly "piney" flavor. Pine nuts are available whole, roasted, baked, ground or pounded into a buttery paste.
- **Walnuts** were the food of royalty in ancient Persia, where their cultivation may have originated. There were walnut groves within the Hanging Gardens of Babylon around 2000 BC. The ancient Greeks and Romans traded walnuts and incorporated them into their mythology. During the Middle Ages, the "Persian" walnut became known as the "English" walnut. Walnuts first came to California via Spanish Franciscan missionaries. In the 1870s, California

walnut agriculture took off in Southern California, near Santa Barbara. Inside a tough shell, a walnut's curly nutmeat halves offer a rich, sweet flavor, and the edible papery skin adds a hint of bitterness to baked goods. Walnuts are available whole (shelled and unshelled), halved and chopped.

Use

- Whole, sliced and slivered almonds are used in both sweet dishes (desserts) and savory dishes (as thickeners for sauces or in stuffing for meats).
- The rich, sweet flavor of hazelnuts and filberts complements coffee and chocolate.
- Versatile pecans add a rich, meaty texture to sweets, baked goods, salads and entrées.
- Once they are shelled and roasted, pine nuts can be added to salads, sauces, candies, cookies and pesto, or can be eaten as a snack. The nuts are standard ingredients in Italian cuisine.
- Toasted, then added in large quantities to breads or cakes, walnuts add a rich color, an interesting texture and a unique flavor. Try our Honeyed Walnut Bread (page 188 or 190).

Nut Flours and Meals

Nut flours and meals are made from very finely ground nuts such as almonds, hazelnuts and pecans. They are not as smooth or as fine as grain flours. Nut flours can be purchased, or you can grind them yourself (see the Technique Glossary, page 301). Don't grind the nuts until you're ready to prepare the recipe. Toast them first for a nuttier flavor. Toasting also dries nut flour, helping to prevent clumping.

- **Almond flour or meal** is made from blanched almonds and is creamy white. Sugar or flour is sometimes added during grinding to absorb the oil from the almonds and prevent clumping, so check purchased almond flour to be sure it is gluten-free. Almond flour can be used in combination with other GF flours in preparing crêpes, pastry and cakes.
- **Hazelnut flour or meal** has a full, rich flavor that is perfect for pastry and anything with orange or chocolate.
- **Pecan flour or meal** is a warm brown, very similar in color to ground flaxseed. It complements recipes made with pumpkin and dried fruits such apricots and dates.

Storage

Store unshelled nuts (including macadamia nuts and pistachios, as well as the nuts listed above) in an airtight container in a cool, dry place for up to 6 months. Refrigerate shelled nuts for up to 6 months. Both shelled and unshelled nuts can be stored in the freezer for up to 1 year. As nuts absorb the flavors of other foods, store them away from foods with strong odors (fish, cabbage, onions). Nuts can become rancid quite quickly if they're exposed to heat, light or humidity during storage. If nuts smell like paint thinner, they are rancid; do not use them.

Refrigerate purchased nut flours and meals for up to 3 months or freeze for up to 1 year.

Nutritional Value

Although the protein is incomplete — except for peanuts (a legume), nuts are deficient in the amino acid lysine — most nuts are rich in potassium and relatively high in iron. Their oil-rich kernels are one of the best vegetable sources of vitamin E; in addition, they supply the B vitamins thiamine, niacin and riboflavin (although roasting can destroy much of the thiamine). They also contain the minerals magnesium, zinc and copper. Almonds, Brazil nuts, hazelnuts and filberts contain good amounts of calcium, and other nuts have at least a small quantity.

Along with these nutrients, however, comes fat, usually a lot of it, which is why nuts are less attractive than legumes or grains as a non-meat protein source. Most of the fat in nuts is unsaturated (and walnuts contain omega-3 fatty acids), but some nuts — especially coconuts, Brazil nuts, macadamias and cashews — contain more saturated fat than the others.

Further Information

- www.bluediamond.com
- www.diamondnuts.com
- www.joyofbaking.com
- www.sunnydayproducts.com

Oats

Rolled oats, also known as oat flakes, were developed in America by the Quaker Oat Company in 1877. Until very recently, celiacs were advised to avoid oats, as they were often contaminated with gluten (from surrounding crops and/or from equipment during processing). In North America, the first crops of pure, uncontaminated oats have now arrived in the marketplace; they are sold as groats (whole oats), rolled oats (oat flakes or oatmeal) and oat flour. Gluten Free Oats of Powell, Wyoming, and Cream Hill Estates of LaSalle, Quebec, are two companies that go through all the steps necessary to eliminate cross-contamination.

Forms of Oats

- "Groats," the whole-grain form of oats, is an old Scottish word that describes an oat kernel with the hull removed. Groats have a sweet, nutty taste with a slight hint of pecan flavor.
- **Rolled oats** (oat flakes or oatmeal) result when groats are steamed and then rolled to flatten. Some rolled oats are also roasted to provide more flavor. These large, separate flakes are also called old-fashioned, thick-cut or porridge oats; they take longer to cook than quick-cooking oats (which are cut into smaller pieces to reduce the cooking time), but they also retain more flavor and nutrition. This is what most people think of as "oatmeal."
- **Oat flour** is made from finely ground groats, which contain much of the bran. Depending on how it is ground, the flour can be almost as nutritious as the whole grain itself (it is heat during grinding that causes nutrient loss). Thanks to its high oil content, oat flour has a sweet, nutty flavor.

Use

- Groats require about 30 minutes to cook. Combine with other grains such as rice, cook and serve instead of potatoes or plain rice.
- Rolled oats can be eaten as a hot breakfast cereal, added to muesli, breads and scones, used to thicken soups and stews or added as a filler or extender to meatloaf and casseroles. Popular uses in North America are in cookies and granolas.
- Oat flour makes baked items moist and more crumbly, but the products stay fresh longer than items baked with wheat flour. Use in quick breads, breads, cookies and cakes.

Introducing Oats to Your Diet

The North American celiac organizations have each taken an individual position on the use of oats in the gluten-free diet:

- The **Gluten Intolerance Group** says, "Research suggests that pure, uncontaminated oats in moderation (1 cup [250 mL] cooked) daily are safe for most persons with celiac disease. . . . work closely with your health care team before deciding to introduce oats in your diet, and . . . have your antibody levels reviewed periodically."
- The **Celiac Disease Foundation** concurs with the Gluten Intolerance Group on all points.
- The **Canadian Celiac Association** recommends a maximum of ½ to ¾ cup (125 to 175 mL) of dry rolled oats per day for adults and ¼ cup (50 mL) for children.
- The **Celiac Sprue Association** recommends excluding oats as the only risk-free choice.

If you decide to add oats to your diet, introduce them gradually. Start with ¼ cup (50 mL) dry rolled oats. If, after a few days, you are tolerating that amount, you can increase your intake to ½ cup (125 mL). Alternate eating ½ cup (125 mL) and ¼ cup (50 mL) per day for several days until you are sure you can tolerate the higher amount. If you can, you can begin to eat ½ cup (125 mL) every day.

Storage
Gluten Free Oats recommends keeping their products refrigerated. Cream Hill Estates says refrigeration is not necessary for their products. In general, groats and rolled oats can be stored in an airtight container in a cool, dry, dark place for up to 2 months or frozen for 6 months. Oat flour can be stored at room temperature for up to 3 months or frozen for up to 6 months.

Nutritional Value
Like all other whole grains, oats supply protein, carbohydrate, dietary fiber, B vitamins, (thiamine, niacin, riboflavin and folate) and minerals (iron, zinc and magnesium). Oats contain a water-soluble form of dietary fiber. Oat fiber reduces the rate of glucose absorption and insulin production after a meal, making it an excellent food for people with diabetes.

Further Information
- www.creamhillestates.com
- www.glutenfreeoats.com
- www.innvista.com

Poppy Seeds

Poppy seeds have been cultivated for over 3,000 years. The Dutch variety, noted for its uniform slate blue color, is recognized as the best-quality seed and comprises most imports into North America. Asian and Indian poppy seeds are typically smaller and are often a creamy beige.

The tiny seeds are kidney-shaped and have a mild, sweet, nutty, dusty flavor. Poppy seeds are available whole or ground. They are most flavorful when roasted and crushed. The hard shell requires a special grinder, so it is more economical to purchase them ground.

Use

- Whole poppy seeds can be sprinkled on top of breads and rolls and added to cakes, cookies, breads and muffins, where they complement orange and lemon flavors. They can also be used to add crunch to sweet and savory dishes, including vegetables and salad dressings.
- Turkish cuisine uses toasted poppy seeds, while Indian and Turkish spice blends rely on crushed poppy seeds for flavor and texture. In India, the smaller beige seed is found in chutneys and is added ground to curry spice mixtures.

Storage

Refrigerate poppy seeds in an airtight container for up to 6 months or freeze for up to 1 year. Because of their high oil content, they tend to go rancid quickly, so purchase in small quantities and taste a few before using.

Nutritional Value

Poppy seeds are high in protein, fat, thiamine and manganese.

Further Information

- www.mccormick.com
- www.nutritiondata.com

Pumpkin Seeds

Pumpkin seeds have long been used in folk medicine and have recently been the subject of a number of studies looking into their health-promoting potential. They are available roasted or raw, salted or unsalted, and with or without hulls. Raw pumpkin seeds without hulls — often known as pepitas ("little seeds" in Spanish) — are a dull, dark olive green. Roasted pumpkin seeds have a rich, almost peanuty flavor.

Use
- Pumpkin seeds can be added to soups, salads, casseroles, yeast breads and quick breads, or they can be ground and used to make sauces.

Storage
Refrigerate pumpkin seeds in an airtight container for up to 6 months or freeze for up to 1 year. Because of their high oil content, they tend to go rancid quickly, so purchase in small quantities and taste a few before using.

Nutritional Value
Pumpkin seeds are packed with protein, fiber, iron, copper, magnesium, manganese and phosphorous.

Further Information
- www.purcellmountainfarms.com
- www.sunnydayproducts.com

Quinoa
The Incas once called quinoa (pronounced *KEEN-wah*) the "mother grain." Beginning with the Spanish conquest in the 1500s, there was a 400-year decline in the production of quinoa. The grain was rediscovered and brought to the U.S. in the 1980s. Peru, Chile and Bolivia cultivate quinoa, referring to it as "little rice." It is now grown in Canada as well. Quinoa is not a true cereal grain but is the fruit of the Chenopodium family and is a relative of Swiss chard, spinach, lamb's-quarters and beets.

Forms of Quinoa
- **Quinoa seeds** are flat with a pointed oval shape and look like a cross between a sesame seed and millet. They are usually pale yellow, but some species vary from almost white through pink, orange or dark red to purple and black. Black quinoa, a rare variety ranging from black to red to yellow, is considered the caviar. Its smaller seed looks interesting in specialty dishes. As quinoa cooks, the outer germ around each grain twists outward, forming a

small, white spiral tail, which is attached to the kernel. The grain itself is soft and delicate, while the tail is crunchy; this creates an interesting texture combination and pleasant "crunch."

- **Quinoa flakes** are whole quinoa kernels rolled flat into flakes of $\frac{1}{8}$ to $\frac{1}{4}$ inch (3 to 5 mm) in diameter.
- **Quinoa flour** is finely ground and tan-colored, with a strong, slightly nutty flavor. Used in small amounts, it results in a product with a tender, moist crumb and good keeping qualities.

Use

- Quinoa seeds have a delicate, almost bland flavor and have been compared to couscous or rice. Although it's lighter, quinoa can be used in any way suitable for rice, or in combination with rice, including pilaf. Cooked quinoa has a fluffy consistency and is excellent as a hot cereal, in casseroles, soups and stews or in stir-fries. It can be eaten as part of a salad, like couscous, or as a cold base similar to tabbouleh. The uncooked seeds may be added instead of barley or rice as a thickener to soups and stews.
- Add quinoa flakes to cookie recipes or use them to replace GF oatmeal or buckwheat flakes in fruit crisp toppings. Flaked quinoa usually takes about 60 to 90 seconds to cook for a hot breakfast cereal.
- Quinoa flour is delicious in baked goods such as pancakes, breads, muffins and crackers. Use in small amounts, as it is strong in flavor. It is perfect in Olive Ciabatta (page 214) and Honey Dijon Toastie (page 216).

Preparation

Before cooking, quinoa seeds must be rinsed to remove their bitter resin-like coating, called saponin. Quinoa is frequently rinsed before it is sold, but rinse again before use to remove any soapy residue that remains. The presence of saponin is obvious by the appearance of soapy-looking "suds" when the seeds are swished in water. Place quinoa seeds in a fine meshed strainer and rinse thoroughly with water. Botanists are now developing saponin-free strains of quinoa.

For information on cooking quinoa, see the Technique Glossary, page 301.

Storage

Store quinoa seeds in an airtight container in a cool, dry, dark place for up to 1 month, refrigerate for up to 6 months or freeze for up to 1 year. Refrigerate cooked quinoa for up to 3 days or freeze for up to 6 months. Store quinoa flakes in a cool, dry place for up to 2 years. Refrigerate quinoa flour for up to 6 months or freeze for up to 1 year.

Nutritional Value

Quinoa is the most nutritious grain available. Like all other whole grains, quinoa supplies protein, carbohydrate, dietary fiber, B vitamins (thiamine, riboflavin, niacin, folate) and minerals (iron, zinc and magnesium). However, it contains more high-quality protein than any other grain and is higher in unsaturated fats and lower in carbohydrate than most. It provides more calcium than milk, as well as phosphorous and vitamin E.

Further Information

- www.quinoa.com
- www.quinoa.net
- www.specialfoods.com
- www.waltonfeed.com

Rice

Rice has been a staple for thousands of years. It is believed that it was first cultivated in central India, but it was quickly adopted by the Chinese. More than 4,500 years later, in the 12th century, it finally reached Europe, and it was brought to the Americas in the 1690s. Today, it is one of the most important food crops in the world.

Types of Rice

- **Long-grain rice** has kernels, or grains, four to five times as long as they are wide. When cooked, it has a soft, fluffy texture, and the kernels stay separate.
- **Medium-grain rice** has a shorter, wider kernel (two to three times as long as it is wide). The cooked grains are more moist and tender than long-grain and have a greater tendency to cling together.
- **Short-grain rice** has a short, plump, almost round kernel. The cooked grains are soft and cling together.

- **White, or "polished," rice**, the most common variety, is available as long-, medium- or short-grain. White rice is refined, with the outer husk, bran and germ removed and the kernel milled until the grain is white.
- **Brown rice** is the whole, unpolished grain of rice, available in long-, medium- and short-grain. It gets its light brown color, nutty flavor and chewy texture from the bran layers. It takes longer to cook than white rice.
- **Converted rice** (parboiled long-grain rice, conditioned, perfected) is a convenient "in-between" rice. The rice is soaked and partially steamed in the husk before the outer bran layer is removed, locking in some of the extra nutrients found in brown rice and giving the uncooked rice a slightly amber color. It has a mild, nutty flavor similar to brown rice, but takes less time to cook.
- **Precooked white or brown rice** has been completely cooked and dehydrated after milling, reducing the time required for cooking.
- **Arborio** (ar-BOH-ree-oh) **rice** gets its name from a village in northern Italy. Its translucent, plump, creamy white short-grain kernels have an opaque white dot at the center. It has the ability to absorb large quantities of liquid, and, when stirred frequently during cooking, develops a creamy texture with a chewy center that absorbs flavors easily. If you want a softer texture and no creaminess, simply cook without stirring. It is done when it is al dente (tender on the outside and firm in the center).
- **Aromatic, or scented, rice** is available in a variety of natural aromas, lengths and colors. The flavor is similar to that of roasted nuts. The most popular forms are:
  - **Basmati rice**, available in both brown and white. It swells only lengthwise when cooked, resulting in long, thin grains (double the length of regular long-grain rice). It has a pungent odor and a strong flavor, and its firm grains stay separate. Northern Indian basmati is considered premium.
  - **Jasmine rice** (Thai jasmine fragrant rice), a long-grain rice available in both brown and white. When cooked, its soft, moist kernels cling together.
  - **Della rice**, a cross between long-grain and basmati developed in the United States. It has an aroma and flavor similar to basmati and cooks dry and separate. The kernels swell in both length and width when cooked.

- **Wild rice** is not technically rice — in fact, it is not even a grain, but a marsh grass seed. It is native to the Great Lakes region of North America and to northern Saskatchewan. The long, shiny, black or dark brown grains take longer to cook than white rice and triple or quadruple in size when cooked. Because of its strong flavor and high price, it is most often eaten in a blend with other rice or grains. In its natural state, wild rice is gluten-free, but when found in boxed wild rice/white rice mixes, it's best avoided.

Use

- Long-grain white or brown rice is suitable for casseroles, Asian-style dishes, fried rice, pilafs and rice salads.
- Choose medium- or short-grain white or brown rice for dishes in which stickier rice is preferred, such as risotto, sushi or rice pudding.
- Replace white rice with brown rice to add variety and nutrition to meals. Its firm texture, flavor and separate grains make it suitable for salad.
- Arborio rice is used mainly in risotto and rice puddings. Its flavor complements asparagus, beets, mushrooms, Parmesan cheese, peas, saffron, shallots, shellfish and veal.
- Basmati rice complements Indian and Middle Eastern dishes such as curry and pilaf.
- Jasmine rice adds an authentic touch to Asian dishes such as stir-fries or red and green curries.
- Wild rice goes well with dishes containing almonds, hazelnuts, wild mushrooms, oranges and pine nuts. Its rich, roasted, smoky, nutty flavor and chewy texture complement wild game, poultry and berries.

Rice is one of the most easily digested grains, which is one reason why rice cereal is often recommended as a baby's first solid.

Cooking Rice

Use the table on page 46 to determine the amounts of rice and liquid to use, as well as cooking times. Combine rice and liquid in a saucepan and bring to a boil. Reduce heat and simmer for the specified time. Remove from heat and let stand, covered, for 5 to 10 minutes, or until all liquid is absorbed. Fluff with a fork.

A serving of cooked rice is $\frac{1}{2}$ cup (125 mL). One pound (500 g) of uncooked rice equals about 2 cups (500 mL) uncooked or 6 cups (1.5 L) cooked.

Rinsing rice or cooking it in excess water then draining results in a loss of water-soluble vitamins and minerals.

Cooking Rice

Uncooked rice (1 cup/250 mL)	Liquid*	Cooking time**	Yield	Additional information
White (long-grain)	1¾–2 cups (425–500 mL)	15–20 minutes	3–4 cups (750 mL–1 L)	
White (medium- or short-grain)	1½–1¾ cups (375–425 mL)	15–20 minutes	3 cups (750 mL)	
Brown	2–2½ cups (500–625 mL)	45–50 minutes	3–4 cups (750 mL–1 L)	
Converted	2–2½ cups (500–625 mL)	20–25 minutes	3–4 cups (750 mL–1 L)	
Arborio***	1½ cups (375 mL)	12–14 minutes	3 cups (750 mL)	Do not rinse.
Basmati	2 cups (500 mL)	12–14 minutes	2 cups (500 mL)	Rinse well before cooking.
Jasmine	1½–2 cups (375–500 mL)	12–15 minutes	2 cups (500 mL)	Rinse well before cooking.
Wild rice	6 cups (1.5 L)	35 minutes uncovered, then 10 minutes covered	3 cups (750 mL)	Rinse well before cooking.

   * Liquid can be water, GF stock or reconstituted GF stock powder
  ** After rice begins to simmer, do not remove the cover and peek. Peeking allows steam to escape, and the rice to become too dry. If rice is not quite tender or liquid is not absorbed after the specified cooking time, replace lid and cook for 2 to 4 minutes longer. Fluff with a fork.
 *** Information applies to steamed Arborio rice. If making risotto, extra liquid and time will be required — see individual recipe.

Rice Flours

- **White rice flour** is produced by grinding uncooked polished rice into a powder that ranges from coarse to very fine. It was once the main flour used in GF baking; however, products made with white rice flour are frequently gritty and crumbly, and they dry out quickly. White rice flour must be used in combination with starches such as corn, potato or tapioca, or a combination of these.
- **Brown rice flour** is milled from the whole grain. It has a grainy texture and provides more fiber and nutrients than white rice flour. It is a creamy brown (only a shade darker than white rice flour) and has a mild, nutty flavor. Brown rice flour results in a product with a grainy texture and a fine, dry crumb. We use it in recipes that require rice flour, including biscuits, breads and cakes.

- **Rice bran** and **rice polish** are the two outer parts of the rice kernel, removed during milling for white rice flour. Rice bran is the outermost layer. When bran and polish are added in small amounts to recipes, the fiber content is increased. Bran and polish are interchangeable in recipes.
- **Sweet rice flour** (glutinous rice flour, mochiko flour, sticky rice flour, mochi flour, sushi rice flour) is made from short-grain rice. It contains more starch than brown or white rice flour. There are two grades: one is beige, grainy and sandy-textured; the other is white, starchy, sticky and less expensive. The latter works better in recipes. It is often used to bread foods before frying or to thicken Asian dishes. It withstands refrigerator and freezer temperatures without separating. We use it to dust baking pans or our fingers for easier handling of sticky dough.
- **Wild rice flour** is gray-brown to black and has a hearty flavor and an interesting texture. It can be added to pancakes, muffins, scones and cookies or used to thicken casseroles, sauces, gravies and stews. Try it in fish, chicken and tempura batters. Best results are achieved when it is mixed with other GF flours.

Storage

Once opened, uncooked white rice can be stored in an airtight container at room temperature. Brown rice should be refrigerated because the bran layers contain oil that could become rancid. Refrigerate cooked rice for up to 7 days or freeze for up to 6 months.

Store rice flours in airtight containers at room temperature for up to 1 year. Refrigerate rice polish and rice bran for up to 6 months or freeze for up to 1 year.

Nutritional Value

Rice is a complex carbohydrate. The protein is considered high quality because it contains all of the essential amino acids. Rice is also a source of thiamine, riboflavin, niacin, phosphorus, selenium and manganese.

Most of the white rice consumed in the United States is enriched with thiamine, niacin and iron (during the milling process, the quantity of these nutrients is reduced). Enriched rice is also fortified with folic acid. Canada, however, does not allow white rice to be enriched.

Brown rice is rich in minerals and vitamins, especially the B complex group. It is a source of unsaturated fat and is the only rice that contains vitamin E. Brown rice is lower in fiber than most other whole grains.

Wild rice has twice the protein and fiber of brown rice.

Rice bran contains thiamine, niacin, vitamin B_6, iron, phosphorus, magnesium, manganese, potassium and fiber.

Further Information
- www.daintyrice.ca
- www.purcellmountainfarms.com
- www.usarice.com
- www.wildfoods.ca

Salba

Salba is a variety of an ancient plant in the mint family called chia (*Salvia hispanica L*), which originated in South America. The Aztecs ground chia into flour to make bread that would sustain them on hunting and trading expeditions and in battle. In the early 1990s, plant breeders in Argentina separated out the few white grains from the mostly black seeds of the chia plant and successfully replanted them to create a white, highly nutritious grain. Today, most Salba is grown in Peru.

Forms of Salba

The name "Salba" is a combination of Salvia and the Latin word for white, "alba."

- **Salba seeds** are flat and oval, similar to sesame seeds in size and shape. They range from off-white through tan to a deeper brown.
- **Ground Salba** is made by grinding seeds in a coffee grinder. Grind only what you can use at one time.
- **Salba gel** is made by combining 1 part ground Salba with 4 parts water, creating a thick gel.

Use
- Salba seeds can be sprinkled on salads, stir-fries, yogurt, oatmeal, cereal and soup.
- Ground Salba can be used to thicken gravies, soups and oatmeal or added to baked goods (use 3 parts flour and 1 part ground Salba).
- Salba gel can be added to cereal, applesauce, yogurt, oatmeal or smoothies, or spread on toast with jam.

Storage

Refrigerate Salba seeds for up to 6 months. Ground Salba and Salba gel should be prepared as needed.

Nutritional Value

Salba is rich in many nutrients, particularly calcium, iron, omega-3 fatty acids and dietary fiber. It provides high-quality protein and is low in sodium. It also contains potassium, magnesium, folate, copper and antioxidants.

Further Information

- www.salba.info

See "Egg-Free Baking" (page 65) for instructions on using Salba to replace eggs in a recipe.

Sesame Seeds

A 4,000-year-old drawing on an Egyptian tomb shows a baker adding sesame seeds to dough. Most of the sesame seeds sold in the United States are grown in Mexico, Central America and China. In some parts of the American South, they are still known as benne, which was sesame's name in Bantu.

The seeds are sold dried, hulled (decorticated) and whole. They are tiny, flat ovals measuring about $\frac{1}{8}$ inch (3 mm) long. Colors include ivory, red, brown, pale gold and black. The flavor is nutty. Black sesame seeds have a more pungent flavor and bitter taste than white or natural sesame seeds. Brown seeds have a nutty, slightly sweet flavor.

Use

- Sesame seeds are used to add texture and flavor to breads, rolls and crackers, and are lightly toasted for salads and salad dressings.
- Middle Eastern, Muslim and Asian seasoning blends use crushed, whole and toasted sesame seeds for flavor and texture.
- Whole raw seeds are ground into the paste tahini, which is used to make many traditional Middle Eastern dishes, such as hummus and the popular Arab appetizer *mezze*.
- Sesame is a key ingredient in halvah, a Middle Eastern confection in which the seeds are ground and pressed into blocks with various sweet or nutty ingredients added.

Storage

Refrigerate sesame seeds in an airtight container for up to 6 months or freeze for up to 1 year. Because of their high oil content, they tend to go rancid quickly, so purchase in small quantities and taste a few before using.

Nutritional Value

Sesame seeds contain protein, fiber, calcium, iron, magnesium, phosphorus, copper, zinc and manganese.

Further Information

- www.mccormick.com
- www.sunnydayproducts.com

Sorghum

Sorghum (also known as milo, great millet, kaffir corn, American broom corn, Guinea corn and jowar) has been grown and eaten by people in Africa and India for thousands of years. It was probably first cultivated in Ethiopia between 4000 and 3000 BC. Ethiopians developed the original white food-grade sorghum to make porridges and flat pancakes. Grain sorghum was known as Guinea corn when it arrived in North America from West Africa with slave traders in the middle of the 19th century.

Sorghum has long, flat leaves with large, feathery seed heads; it looks very similar to a corn plant but is shorter and more colorful. White food-grade sorghum has white oval berries with tan husks and produces a gray-tan flour.

Forms of Sorghum

One of the largest snack chip makers in Japan is test-marketing a product made from sorghum in Tokyo convenience stores. Researchers hope to create a quick breakfast food for those with gluten intolerance, especially children.

- **Sorghum grains (seeds)** are smaller than peppercorns but have a hearty, chewy texture and a slightly sweet, nutty, earthy taste. The kernels can be extruded, steam-flaked, popped, or puffed and micronized. Sorghum should not be used as a sprouting grain as the young shoots are very poisonous.
- **Sorghum flour** tends to be coarser in texture than many GF flours, as the most common form is stone-ground. The most wheat-like of all GF flours, it is the best general-purpose flour, giving baked items a warm, creamy color. Because its flavor is neutral, it absorbs other flavors well.
- **Sorghum syrup** is a molasses-like sweetener that is not as popular today as it once was.

Use

- Whole-grain sorghum is commonly used to make porridges, tortillas and rice substitute. It is also sold popped, just like popcorn.
- Puffed sorghum is used in snacks, granola cereals, granola bars, baked products and dry snack cakes, and is added to soups as a GF substitute for couscous, bulgur and pearled barley.
- Cracked sorghum is used in legume and/or vegetable mixtures.
- Sorghum flour adds protein to home-baked goods such as scones, cakes, cookies, breads, muffins, pizza dough, waffles, cereals, energy bars, salty snack foods, pastas and Indian chapati (an unleavened flatbread).

Preparation

To cook whole-grain sorghum, first sort and rinse the seeds. Soak 1 cup (250 mL) overnight in 3 cups (750 mL) of water. Simmer for 45 to 60 minutes, or until tender.

We recently purchased sorghum flour from a variety of sources, only to find that consistency varies. We recommend sifting twice before measuring.

Storage

Store sorghum grain and flour in airtight containers in a cool, dry, dark place for up to 1 month, refrigerate for up to 6 months or freeze for up to 1 year.

Nutritional Value

Like all other whole grains, sorghum supplies protein, carbohydrate, dietary fiber, B vitamins (thiamine, niacin, riboflavin, folate) and minerals (iron, zinc and magnesium). Sorghum flour contains both insoluble fiber and smaller amounts of soluble fiber, as well as phosphorous, potassium and vitamin B_6.

The protein and starch in sorghum endosperm are more slowly digested than those in other grains, making it beneficial for people with diabetes. Some sorghum varieties are so rich in antioxidants, which protect against cell damage, that they are comparable to blueberries (known for their high antioxidant levels).

Rather than using a standard mix of flours in our recipes, we like to vary the proportions of flours and starches so that each recipe has a unique flavor and texture. We love the results we get when we use a mixture of sorghum flour and bean flour with strong flavors such as pumpkin, chocolate, molasses, dates and rhubarb.

Further Information

- www.csaceliacs.org
- www.innvista.com
- www.recipetips.com
- www.sorghumgrowers.com

Soy

"Soy" (soya, soybean or glycine max) refers to soybeans and the products made from them. Soybeans have been cultivated in China for over 5,000 years. They were brought to the United States as ballast in marine vessels, and dried soybeans were used as "coffee" during the Civil War. Soybeans are often called the "golden crop" because of their many by-products, used in food, feed and industrial products.

Forms of Soy

- **Soybeans** are the only beans to contain all of the amino acids needed to make a complete protein, just like meat. Cooked soaked soybeans have a "beany" flavor; however, blanching destroys an enzyme responsible for that flavor. Some people find soybeans indigestible and bitter.
- **Soy flour** is made by grinding roasted whole dry soybeans into a fine powder. It is often dry-roasted after grinding to improve flavor and digestibility. Soy flour is available in full-fat (natural), low-fat and defatted versions. Full-fat soy flour contains the natural oils found in the soybean; defatted soy flour has had the oils removed during processing. Soy flour is yellowy gold; the higher the fat, the deeper the color. It has a pungent, nutty, slightly bitter flavor that is enhanced by the flavors of accompanying flours. It has a strong odor when wet, but this "bakes off." It is widely used by the food industry to make moist, tender baked goods that stay fresh longer.
- **Tofu** (soybean curd) is made by curdling soy beverage (see "Lactose-Free Milk Substitutes," page 62) in a process similar to making cheese. Because it has a bland, spongy texture, tofu absorbs the flavor of other foods when you marinate or cook it, making it versatile and easily digested. Regular tofu (cotton or momen), sold in water-filled packs, is the most common. Silken tofu (kinugoshi), made from extra-thick soy beverage, is a creamy, custard-like product. It contains less water than regular and does not have to be

> Studies have shown that 15% of celiacs cannot tolerate soybeans or soy products.

pressed. Tofu is available in a variety of textures. The type and degree of firmness you choose will be based on what you intend to use it for (see "Use," below). Do not substitute one for another.

Use

- Fresh soybean pods (edamame) can be eaten as a vegetable.
- Soy flour adds rich color, fine texture, a pleasant nutty flavor, tenderness and moistness to baked goods. Products containing soy flour bake faster and tend to brown quickly, so the baking time may need to be shortened or the oven temperature lowered. Tenting baked goods with foil partway through the baking time also helps.
- Soy flour can also be used to thicken sauces and gravies, to add a nutty flavor and protein boost to pancake batter and to enrich pasta and breakfast cereals. Added to fried foods such as donuts, soy flour reduces the amount of fat absorbed by the dough.
- Puréed silken tofu is used to replace higher-fat lactose-containing dairy products such as cream cheese (in cheesecake), cream (in creamed soups), sour cream (in dips) or mayonnaise (in creamy salad dressings).
- Soft tofu is good for recipes that call for blended tofu. Its texture is similar to that of al dente pasta. Use it for sauces, dips and salad dressings.
- Medium-firm tofu is an excellent general-purpose product.
- Firm and extra-firm tofu are higher in protein, fat and calcium than other forms. They are thick, dense and solid and can be sliced, cubed or diced. Choose for cheesecakes and puddings, for grilling, for use in stir-fries or as a meat alternative in salads, stews, soups and casseroles.

> 12 oz (340 g) shelf-stable packaged silken tofu = 1½ cups (375 mL) puréed tofu.

Storage

Store dried soybeans in a dry, airtight container at room temperature for up to 1 year.

Refrigerate full-fat soy flour for up to 6 months or freeze for up to 1 year. Defatted soy flour has a longer shelf life because the germ, including the oil, has been removed; store it in an airtight container at room temperature for up to 1 year.

Usually located in the produce section, regular tofu must be refrigerated and used before the expiry date. It can be frozen for up to 1 month. Leftover tofu should be covered with fresh water and stored in the refrigerator. Change the water daily.

(Water keeps the tofu from drying out or absorbing the flavor of other foods.)

Shelf-stable silken tofu has a shelf life of up to 1 year; however, once opened, it should be refrigerated and used within 2 days. Silken tofu can also be frozen for up to 5 months. The texture becomes firmer and chewier, and the tofu absorbs more flavor after it is thawed.

Nutritional Value

Soy flour is a source of high-quality protein, containing almost three times as much protein as wheat flour (depending on the type used: full-fat has 35% protein content; defatted has 50%). It also provides fiber, iron, calcium, magnesium, B vitamins (riboflavin, folate and pantothenic acid) and phytochemicals (a group of compounds that may help prevent chronic diseases). Fat content ranges from 20% for full-fat to 1% for defatted.

Further Information
- http://chinesefood.about.com
- www.innvista.com
- www.recipetips.com
- www.soya.be
- www.soyfoods.com
- www.sunrise-soya.com
- www.talksoy.com
- http://vegetarian.about.com

Starches

The endosperm, which makes up the largest part of any grain, is mainly a complex carbohydrate called starch. Starches have two purposes in gluten-free baking: to lighten baked products and to thicken liquids for sauces or gravies.

Types of Starches

Arrowroot biscuits are one of the first foods given to babies, as they are very easily digested. They're good for the older population — including those with illness — too.

- **Arrowroot** (arrowroot starch, arrowroot powder, arrowroot starch flour) is made from the root of the arrowroot plant. It is a fine, white, tasteless starchy powder with a mild aroma. Arrowroot is more expensive and may be more difficult to find than other starches. (Cornstarch can be substituted one to one in any recipe where arrowroot is used as a thickener.) Arrowroot thickens liquids almost immediately at a lower temperature than either cornstarch or wheat flour. Due to its greater thickening ability, use only half as much arrowroot as wheat flour. Its consistency does not hold as long after cooking.

- **Cornstarch** (corn flour, maize corn flour, *crème de maïs*) is made from a high-starch variety of corn. It is a fine, white, tasteless starchy powder that is used as a thickening agent. Cornstarch doesn't thicken well when mixed with acidic liquids such as lemon juice. Sauces made with cornstarch turn spongy when frozen. Cornstarch has twice the thickening power of wheat flour.
- **Potato starch** (potato starch flour) is often confused with potato flour, but one cannot be substituted for the other. Potato starch is made from only the starch of potatoes, and is therefore less expensive than potato flour. It is a very fine, silky, white powder with a bland taste. It lumps easily and must be sifted frequently. To make gravy without adding fat, use potato starch, as it thickens when heated with larger amounts of liquid in a saucepan.

A permitted ingredient for Passover (unlike cornstarch and other grain-based foods), potato starch is often found with kosher products in supermarkets.

- **Potato flour** is made from the whole potato, including the skin. Because it has been cooked, it absorbs large amounts of water. Potato flour is much denser and heavier than potato starch and has a definite potato flavor. Potato flour mixes well in cold water, cooks quickly without lumps and turns transparent after heating. Potato flour is always used in very small quantities. For thickening, use 2 tsp (10 mL) for every cup (250 mL) of liquid.
- **Tapioca** comes from the root of the cassava plant. It is available as starch (flour), pellets (called pearl tapioca), granules and flakes. All forms are brilliant white and swell into a pale, translucent jelly to thicken the liquid in which they are cooked.

If you plan to freeze a dish, use tapioca starch, as it remains stable when frozen.

- **Tapioca starch** (tapioca flour, tapioca starch flour, cassava flour, yucca starch, manioc, manihot or *almidon de yucca*) is powdery fine, white and mildly sweet. It thickens quickly when heated with water, and at a lower temperature than cornstarch, so it can be added to sauces at the last minute. Some don't like using it to thicken sauces, stews and soups because of its glossy appearance.
- **Pearl tapioca** looks like small, uneven, milky white balls and is used to make pudding. It comes in several sizes and in regular and instant forms. Regular pearl tapioca requires longer soaking and yields larger lumps than instant tapioca. Instant (quick-cooking) tapioca resembles small white beads and is used to thicken pie fillings.

Use

- Use arrowroot as a thickener only when a shiny gloss is desired, as it can look unnatural in a gravy or meat sauce. Common in Chinese cuisine, it is used to thicken soups, stir-fries and gravies, in clear glazes for fruit pies and in clear fruit sauces. It should not be used to thicken dairy-based sauces, as it turns them slimy. When mixed with GF flours to make breads, cookies and pastries, arrowroot helps the baked goods bind better and lightens the finished product.
- Use cornstarch to thicken sauces, gravies, soups, stews, cream fillings, custards and puddings. Cornstarch helps prevent eggs from curdling in custards and causes heat to be transmitted more evenly throughout. When mixed with GF flours to make breads, cookies and pastries, cornstarch helps the baked goods bind better and lightens the finished product.
- Potato starch can be used to thicken soups, gravies and sauces. When combined with other GF flours, it adds moistness to baked goods and gives them a light and airy texture. It also causes breads to rise higher.
- Potato flour is not used like other flours in baking as it would absorb too much liquid and make the product gummy. Small amounts are used to hold the product together. Use it in potato-based recipes to enhance the potato flavor or to thicken soups, gravies, and sauces. Potato flour can be added in very small quantities to breads, puddings and cakes. We rarely use potato flour (Shirley's Old-Fashioned Donuts, page 282, and Cinnamon Buns, page 228, are the exceptions), but we frequently use potato starch.
- Tapioca starch gives a transparent high gloss to fruits and makes a perfectly smooth filling. It's the perfect product to use with high-acid fruits. It is used to thicken soups, glazes, puddings, custards, sauces and juicy fruit pie fillings. Tapioca starch lightens baked goods and gives them a slightly sweet, chewy texture.

Using Starches as Thickeners

- To thicken using arrowroot, mix it with an equal amount of cold water, and then whisk the slurry into a hot liquid for about 30 seconds. Bring the liquid to a boil to eliminate

Thickener Substitutions

Starches	To thicken 1 cup (250 mL) of liquid	Cooking precautions	Cooked appearance	Tips
Arrowroot	2 tbsp (25 mL)	• add during last 5 minutes of cooking • stir only occasionally • do not boil	• clear shine • glossier than cornstarch	• thickens at a lower temperature than cornstarch • not as firm as cornstarch when cool • doesn't break down as quickly as cornstarch • more expensive • separates when frozen
Cornstarch	2 tbsp (25 mL)	• stir constantly • boil gently for only 1 to 3 minutes	• translucent and shiny	• thickens as it cools • boiling too rapidly causes thinning • boiling for more than 7 minutes causes thinning • add acid (lemon juice) after removing from heat
Potato starch	1 tbsp (15 mL)	• stir constantly	• more translucent and clearer than cornstarch	• lumps easily • thickest at boiling point • thickens as it cools • separates when frozen
Tapioca starch (cassava)	3 tbsp (45 mL)	• add during last 5 minutes of cooking • stir constantly	• transparent and shiny	• dissolves more easily than cornstarch • firms more as it cools • best to use for freezing

Flours	To thicken 1 cup (250 mL) of liquid	Cooking precautions	Cooked appearance	Tips
Amaranth flour	3 tbsp (45 mL)	• browns quickly and could burn if not watched carefully • thickens at boiling point and slightly more after 5 to 7 minutes of boiling • reheats in microwave	• golden brown color • cloudy, opaque • smooth	• nutty, beefy aroma • if too thick, can be thinned with extra liquid • reheats • excellent for gravy
Bean flour	3 tbsp (45 mL)	• thickens after 2 to 3 minutes of boiling • does not thicken more with extra cooking	• warm tan color • cloudy, opaque • smooth	• can be used for sauces • brown in hot fat to a golden color
Rice flour (brown or white)	2 tbsp (25 mL)	• dissolve in cold liquid rather than hot fat or pan drippings • thickens after 5 to 7 minutes of boiling • continues to thicken with extra cooking	• opaque, cloudy • grainy texture • bland flavor	• thickens more as it cools • thickens rapidly when reheated and stirred • stable when frozen
Sorghum flour	2 tbsp (25 mL)	• thickens after 2 to 3 minutes of boiling • does not thicken more with extra cooking	• dull • similar to wheat flour	• thickens as it cools • reheats well on stovetop or in microwave • thickens quickly when extra is added
Sweet rice flour	2 tbsp (25 mL)	• thickens after 5 to 8 minutes of boiling	• shiny, opaque • grainy texture • bland flavor	• thickens as it cools

the chalky white appearance and starchy taste. Arrowroot begins to thicken before the boiling point, but doesn't lose its thickening ability when accidentally boiled a little bit too long. The finished product looks transparent, almost clear, like a high-gloss gel.

- To avoid lumps, cornstarch must be dissolved in an equal amount of cold water before it is added to hot liquids. (Mixing it with a granular solid such as granulated sugar also disperses it into a liquid.) Bring the liquid to a boil to eliminate the cloudy white appearance and starchy taste, then reduce the heat to medium or medium-low and cook, stirring gently, for 1 minute only. Don't overcook, or use too high a temperature, or the sauce will break down and thin out.
- For best thickening results, mix potato starch with twice the amount of cold water before adding it to hot liquids. Liquids thickened with potato starch should never be boiled, or the thickening ability will be lost. Sauce thickened using potato starch becomes watery again when cooled.

Storage

Arrowroot starch, cornstarch, potato starch, potato flour, tapioca starch and pearl tapioca can be stored in airtight, moisture-proof containers in a cool, dark place for an indefinite length of time.

Nutritional Value

Arrowroot, cornstarch, potato starch and tapioca starch are all high in carbohydrate.

Further Information

Arrowroot
- www.glutenfreemall.com
- www.innvista.com
- www.recipetips.com

Cornstarch
- www.innvista.com
- www.recipetips.com

Potato Starch
- www.foodsubs.com
- www.recipetips.com

Tapioca Starch
- www.innvista.com
- www.jodelibakery.netfirms.com

Sunflower Seeds

Sunflower seeds come from the center of the tall, daisy-like sunflower, which is native to North America. The plump, nut-like kernels grow in teardrop shapes within gray-and-white shells. They are sold raw and roasted, salted, seasoned and plain. Shelled sunflower seeds are sometimes labeled "sunflower kernels" or "sunflower nutmeats." When buying seeds in-shell, look for clean, unbroken shells. Be sure the seeds are crisp and fresh, not limp, rubbery or off-tasting.

Use
- Sunflower seeds can be added to baked goods, sprinkled on a salad or nibbled as a snack. We prefer the shelled, unroasted (raw), unsalted ones for yeast breads baked in a bread machine. If only roasted, salted seeds are available, rinse under hot water and dry well before using.

Storage
Refrigerate sunflower seeds in an airtight container for up to 6 months or freeze for up to 1 year. Because of their high oil content, they tend to go rancid quickly, so purchase in small quantities and taste a few before using.

Nutritional Value
Sunflower seeds are an outstanding source of the antioxidant vitamin E and also supply good amounts of thiamine and other B vitamins, as well as minerals including copper, magnesium, manganese and selenium.

Further Information
- www.sunnydayproducts.com

Teff

Teff (tef, lovegrass, annual bunch grass, Ethiopian millet), a staple crop of Ethiopia, is believed to have originated as a foraged wild grass with the ancient civilizations of Abyssinia, in Ethiopia, between 4000 and 1000 BC. Teff seeds were discovered in a pyramid thought to date back to 3359 BC. The name "teff" is derived from the Amharic word *teffa*, which means "lost" (because the grain is small, it is easily lost when dropped). Teff arrived in the United States in the 1980s and is currently being introduced into the diet of North Americans. It is related to millet.

Forms of Teff

- **Teff grain** is the smallest grain in the world, tinier than a poppy seed and only twice the size of the period at the end of this sentence. Depending on the variety, the seeds can be white, ivory or brown. Brown teff has a subtle hazelnut, almost chocolate-like flavor; white teff has a chestnut-like flavor; ivory teff has a mild, slightly molasses-like sweetness and nutty taste. The darker varieties are earthier-tasting.
- **Teff flour** milled from brown teff has a sweet, nutty flavor, while flour from white teff is milder.

A hundred and fifty teff seeds weigh as much as one kernel of wheat; seven grains will fit onto the head of a pin.

Use

- The grain can be sprouted to use in salads and sandwiches.
- Raw teff grain can substitute for some of the seeds, nuts or other small grains in recipes. Due to its small size, use only ½ cup (125 mL) of teff to replace 1 cup (250 mL) of sesame seeds.
- Teff grain is a good thickener for soups, stews and gravies.
- Use teff grain in stir-fry dishes and casseroles and to make grain burgers. Cook it to make breakfast porridge, a polenta-like side dish, stuffing or pilaf. It can be cooked alone or in combination with other grains and vegetables. It combines well with brown rice, millet, kasha (toasted buckwheat groats) and cornmeal. Cooked teff can be seasoned with cinnamon, ginger, garlic, cardamom, chilies, basil or cilantro.
- Ethiopians use teff as the main ingredient in their staple bread, injera. Teff grain is ground into flour, fermented for three days and made into a thin, sourdough-type flatbread that complements the spices in their food. Used to scoop up meat and vegetable stews, injera also lines the tray on which the stews are served, soaking up their juices as the meal progresses. When this edible tablecloth is eaten, the meal is officially over.

- Teff flour has excellent baking qualities. Use in breads, quick breads, pancakes, waffles, pie crusts, gingerbread, crackers and cookies.
- Teff flour is a good thickener for soups, stews, gravies and puddings.

Like rice, teff cooks quickly. Cook just long enough to open the grain. For extra flavor, toast the grains first.

Storage

Store teff grain and flour in airtight containers in a cool, dry, dark place for up to 1 month, refrigerate for up to 6 months or freeze for up to 1 year. Cooked teff grain can be stored, covered, in the refrigerator for up to 3 days or frozen for up to 6 months.

Nutritional Value

In teff, the germ and the bran (where nutrients concentrate) make up almost the whole grain. Because it is so small, there is no way to remove the husk, bran and germ, which means that none of the nutrients are lost when the grain is ground into flour. Like all other whole grains, teff supplies protein, carbohydrate, dietary fiber, B vitamins, (thiamine, niacin, riboflavin, folate) and minerals (iron, zinc and magnesium). Teff is much higher in iron and calcium than wheat, rice, millet or oats. Though not a complete protein like quinoa, it has an excellent amino acid composition, with more lysine (the amino acid most often deficient in grain) than barley, millet or wheat and only slightly less than rice or oats.

Further Information
- www.hort.purdue.edu/newcrop
- www.innvista.com
- www.recipetips.com
- www.teffco.com

Lactose Intolerance

Lactose is a natural sugar found in milk and milk products. Almost all milk, including cow's milk and goat's milk, contains lactose. Lactase, an enzyme made within the digestive tract, is needed to digest lactose into two simpler sugars the body can use. When not enough lactase is made, lactose is not broken down and abdominal pain, bloating and diarrhea result. This inability to digest lactose is called lactose intolerance or lactase deficiency. The symptoms vary among individuals.

Sources of Lactose

Major sources of lactose in the diet include cow's milk and goat's milk — whether non-fat or whole, in liquid or in powdered form — and products made from milk, including cottage cheese, cream, yogurt, buttermilk, butter, sour cream and ice cream.

Hidden sources may include sausages and wieners, commercial baking mixes, snacks and cookies, and other commercially prepared products. Lactose itself is not listed on food labels, but look for lactic acid, lactalbumin, lactate, calcium compounds or casein.

> Parve foods do not contain dairy products. Other kosher products may or may not have dairy in them — read the label.

A Lactose-Free Diet

All milk products do not contain the same amount of lactose. The processes that turn milk into yogurt and hard cheese (including Parmesan, mozzarella, Swiss and aged Cheddar) lower the lactose level, and these items may be digestible even for those with lactose intolerance. Look for yogurt containing an active or live culture.

When developing the lactose-free recipes in this book, we discovered many excellent products on the market. Below are a few we used, but there are others. Check labels and with manufacturers to be sure your choices are also gluten-free. Many manufacturers have lactose-free products listed on their websites.

Lactose-Free Milk Substitutes

- **Soy beverage** (fortified soy beverage, soy milk) has a sweet, nutty flavor and is more easily digested than cow's milk but should not be used as a substitute in infant formulas. Fresh soy beverage is sold plain and flavored and in full-fat, reduced-fat and fat-free forms. Keep it refrigerated in its original container and use before the best-before date. It needs to be shaken well every time it is used, as it settles. Soy beverage sold in an aseptic (shelf-stable) package can be kept at room temperature for up to 1 year; after opening, it needs to be refrigerated and should be used within 1 week. Freezing is not recommend (it can be frozen, but upon defrosting it tends to separate).

Because of soy beverage's bland flavor, baked goods made with it may need more seasonings. Soy beverage can be used to replace milk cup for cup (mL for mL) in milkshakes, puddings, soups and creamy sauces. Use soy beverage instead of evaporated milk to make lower-fat custards, cream sauces and pumpkin pies.

Soy beverage is a good source of protein and, unlike cow's milk, contains fiber, is low in saturated fat and is cholesterol-free. It is a good source of isoflavones (though not as good a source as soybeans themselves or tofu). Since eliminating milk and milk products from the diet also eliminates a major source of calcium, look for a soy beverage that is fortified with calcium and vitamins A, D2, B_{12} and riboflavin.

- **Soy powder** (soy milk powder) is used to make liquid soy beverage to substitute for cow's milk in baking recipes. It can be added with the dry ingredients or reconstituted with 4 cups (1 L) water for each 1 cup (250 mL) powder.
- **Coconut milk, rice milk and almond milk** are non-soy-based lactose-free products.
- **Lactose-free milk** can be found in refrigerated containers near the regular cow's milk. There are several brands on the market, available in different levels of fat.

Lactose-Free Yogurt Substitutes

Yogurt containing an active bacterial culture is more easily digested than other dairy products. However, if you can't tolerate dairy yogurt, soy yogurt has a similar texture and consistency. It is available plain and in a variety of flavors. Soy yogurt must be refrigerated and used before the best-before date. We found it held well, and we were able to use some and store the rest for later. It did not become thin and watery. Enjoy it in both dips and baking.

To make lactose-free buttermilk, add 1 tsp (5 mL) lemon juice or vinegar to 1 cup (250 mL) fortified soy beverage or lactose-free milk and let stand for 5 minutes. You can also substitute $1/2$ cup (125 mL) soft tofu blended with $1/3$ cup (75 mL) water for 1 cup (250 mL) buttermilk.

Lactose-Free Cheese Substitutes

Many hard cheeses, such as aged Cheddar and Parmesan, are very low in lactose, and some people with lactose intolerance can tolerate them. If you're not one of them, there are a variety of lactose-free cheeses on the market, including soy cheese and rice Cheddar and mozzarella.

Soy cheese (firm and soft) is a cheese substitute made from soy beverage. Check the label carefully, as some commercial soy cheese may also contain lactose. The firm cheese can be used as you would dairy cheese, although it does not melt the same. Firm soy cheese is often colored and/or flavored to resemble feta, mozzarella or Cheddar. Soy cheese slices are available in individually wrapped packages as mozzarella, American and roasted garlic. Spread soft soy cheese on GF toast or use it in a dip.

Lactose-Free Cream Cheese and Sour Cream Substitutes

Plain soy yogurt or soft soy cheese can substitute for sour cream or cream cheese. There is also a lactose-free sour cream on the market.

Lactose-Free Fat Substitutes

We found a variety of buttery spreads and lactose-free margarines that worked well in baking. Read the label carefully, though, as several buttery spreads contain lactose. These spreads soften quickly, directly out of the refrigerator, so they do not need to be brought to room temperature before use in baking. Be careful not to cream them too long with a mixer, or they could become watery.

Further Information

- www.neilsondairy.com
- www.sonice.ca
- www.sunrise-soya.com
- www2.texaschildrenshospital.org/internetarticles/uploadedfiles/324.pdf

Egg-Free Baking

When we were developing recipes for this book, we wanted to have egg-free variations for as many recipes as possible. We were hesitant at first, as we have long been aware of the versatile roles played by eggs in the baking process — they are used for leavening or lightness, and as a binder to help hold baked goods together. However, we forged ahead. We first developed the recipe — for example, a muffin — with eggs, then chose an egg substitute based on the purpose of the eggs in the recipe and the flavor and texture of the specific muffin. Once we were satisfied with the recipe, we passed both the original and the egg-free samples on to our taste-testers, without telling them which was which. Many times, they preferred the egg-free version.

Not all recipes are suitable for egg substitutions. Some recipes, including several of our bread machine yeast breads, Stollen (page 226) and Carol's Brownies (page 276), which requires several eggs, presented a challenge, and we were unhappy with the results when we tried to substitute for eggs. The Rum and Pecan Pie (page 245) and the Mango and Ginger Cream Tart (page 246) required eggs as custard, so we were unable to develop what we felt were acceptable egg-free variations.

Here are some of the ways we developed egg-free variations for you.

Ground Flaxseed

You'll be pleasantly surprised, as we were, when you use ground flaxseed to replace eggs in baking recipes. The ground flaxseed you use can be flax flour, milled flaxseed, sprouted flax flour or grind-your-own flaxseed. When you combine it with warm water and let it stand for at least 5 minutes, it forms a thick gel, about the consistency of a raw egg white.

We did not stick to a set replacement formula in our recipes. In many, each egg was replaced with 2 tbsp (25 mL) ground flaxseed and 1/4 cup (50 mL) warm tap water. However, this needed to be adjusted in some recipes to create a great product similar to the original. We like to add the gel with the liquid ingredients while the mixer is running. When using a bread machine, we add the gel to the bread machine baking pan with the other liquids.

Baked goods made with ground flaxseed tend to brown more quickly than those made with eggs and sometimes need to be tented with foil to prevent burning. However, many require an extra couple of minutes of baking time to reach the 200°F (100°C) desired. The baked product rises slightly higher, browns more and is lighter in texture, with a slightly nuttier taste. It does not become dry and crumbly but stays moist when frozen.

Ground Salba

In several recipes, we substituted ground Salba in the same amounts as ground flaxseed. Grind Salba even finer than flaxseed, or the product could be slightly gritty. When mixed with warm water in the same proportions, Salba forms a thicker gel.

Commercial Egg Replacer

The egg substitutes sold in most supermarkets contain egg products and should not be confused with commercial egg replacer. Egg replacer is a white powder containing a combination of baking powder and starches. It is added with the dry ingredients so that it is well mixed in before it touches the liquids. The oil or other fat in the recipe may have to be increased slightly. We used egg replacer in recipes where we wanted a white product and did not want the slightly nutty taste contributed by ground flaxseed.

These are the products we used to replace eggs in baking. There are others you might like to try. Explore the websites below for additional suggestions.

Further Information

- www.ener-g.com
- www.glutenfree.com
- www.kingsmill.com
- www.pioneerthinking.com
- www.sunrise-soya.com
- www.vegcooking.com

Dips, Beverages, Soups and Salads

Garlicky Feta Spinach Dip

**Makes 1½ cups
(375 mL)
(1 tbsp/15 mL
per serving)**

This dip, with the Mediterranean flavors of garlic, oregano, rosemary and marjoram, is perfect served with bread cubes or as a dip for veggies. Keep some in the refrigerator for when neighbors drop in.

Tips

We recommend rinsing spinach under cold running water, even though it is labeled as washed.

If you can only find unflavored feta, add 1 to 2 cloves minced garlic and fresh or dried oregano, rosemary and marjoram to taste.

½	package (10 oz/300 g) fresh spinach (about 5 cups/1.25 L), trimmed	½
3 oz	Mediterranean-flavored lactose-free soy feta or feta cheese	90 g
2	green onions, coarsely chopped	2
½ cup	GF lactose-free mayonnaise or GF mayonnaise	125 mL
½ cup	lactose-free plain yogurt or plain yogurt	125 mL

1. In a microwave-safe bowl, microwave spinach, uncovered, on High for 2 to 3 minutes, stirring halfway through, until spinach is just wilted. Squeeze out excess moisture.

2. In a food processor fitted with a metal blade, pulse spinach, feta, green onions, mayonnaise and yogurt, scraping down sides occasionally, until smooth.

3. Transfer to a bowl, cover and refrigerate for at least 2 hours to allow flavors to develop and blend. Store in the refrigerator for up to 2 weeks.

Variations

Substitute baby spinach for the spinach, and ⅓ cup (75 mL) chopped fresh chives for the green onions.

Substitute kale or Swiss chard for the spinach and microwave until wilted

NUTRITIONAL VALUE per serving	
Calories	41
Fat, total	4 g
Fat, saturated	0 g
Cholesterol	5 mg
Sodium	38 mg
Carbohydrate	1 g
Fiber	0 g
Protein	1 g
Calcium	15 mg
Iron	0 mg

Sun-Dried Tomato Bacon Dip

We cleaned out the refrigerator one day and developed the recipe for this dip, which has become a personal favorite to serve with fresh vegetables.

Tip

Use dry, not oil-packed, sun-dried tomatoes in recipes.

¼ cup	lactose-free soy cream cheese or cream cheese, softened	50 mL
¼ cup	lactose-free plain yogurt or plain yogurt	50 mL
¼ cup	snipped sun-dried tomatoes	50 mL
3	slices GF bacon, cooked crisp and crumbled	3
¼ cup	packed fresh cilantro, snipped	50 mL

1. In a small bowl, combine cream cheese and yogurt. Stir in sun-dried tomatoes, bacon and cilantro until well combined. Cover and refrigerate for at least 2 hours to allow flavors to develop and blend. Store in the refrigerator for up to 2 weeks.

Variations

Substitute lactose-free sour cream or sour cream for the yogurt.

For a milder flavor, use half parsley and half cilantro.

Vary the fresh herb — try substituting basil or dill for the cilantro.

NUTRITIONAL VALUE per serving	
Calories	31
Fat, total	3 g
Fat, saturated	1 g
Cholesterol	1 mg
Sodium	56 mg
Carbohydrate	1 g
Fiber	0 g
Protein	1 g
Calcium	3 mg
Iron	0 mg

Crispy Sesame Wafers

**Makes 42 wafers
(1 per serving)**

Enjoy this rich, savory sesame wafer with a salad or soup!

Tips

For information on toasting seeds, see the Technique Glossary, page 301.

Watch these carefully during baking — even as little as 1 minute too long can cause the bottoms to burn.

♦ *Preheat oven to 325°F (160°C)*
♦ *Baking sheets, lined with parchment paper*

⅓ cup	soy flour	75 mL
¼ tsp	GF baking powder	1 mL
1 cup	sesame seeds, toasted	250 mL
2 tsp	anise seeds	10 mL
2 tsp	caraway seeds	10 mL
2 tsp	fennel seeds	10 mL
½ cup	lactose-free margarine or margarine	125 mL
¼ cup	granulated sugar	50 mL
¼ cup	water	50 mL

1. In a large bowl or plastic bag, combine soy flour, baking powder, sesame, anise, caraway and fennel seeds. Mix well and set aside.

2. In a separate bowl, using an electric mixer, cream margarine and sugar. Add water and beat until well blended. Slowly beat in dry ingredients until just combined.

3. Drop by small spoonfuls, at least 2 inches (5 cm) apart, onto prepared baking sheets. Flatten with a moistened flat-bottomed drinking glass. Bake in preheated oven for 13 to 16 minutes, or until lightly browned. Let cool on baking sheet for 2 to 3 minutes. Transfer to a rack and let cool completely. Store in an airtight container for up to 3 weeks.

NUTRITIONAL VALUE per serving	
Calories	52
Fat, total	2 g
Fat, saturated	0 g
Cholesterol	0 mg
Sodium	30 mg
Carbohydrate	2 g
Fiber	0 g
Protein	1 g
Calcium	8 mg
Iron	5 mg

Variations

Substitute ½ cup (125 mL) untoasted flaxseed or poppy seeds for half of the sesame seeds.

For a mild-flavored wafer, substitute 2 tbsp (25 mL) flaxseed or poppy seeds for the anise, caraway and fennel seeds.

Berry Smoothie

Makes 1 to 2 servings

Berries are a powerhouse of nutrition. Try our smooth, thick and refreshing smoothie for breakfast on the move.

Tip

There's no need to thaw the berries. Frozen berries add a thick texture to the smoothie.

10	frozen blackberries	10
5	frozen strawberries	5
½ cup	crushed pineapple, including juice	125 mL
½ cup	fortified strawberry-flavored soy beverage	125 mL
1 tbsp	liquid honey	15 mL
½ tsp	vanilla	2 mL

1. In a blender or food processor, purée blackberries, strawberries, pineapple, soy beverage, honey and vanilla until smooth. Serve immediately.

Variations

Substitute 10 to 15 raspberries or ⅓ cup (75 mL) blueberries for the blackberries, or use a combination of all three.

Substitute fruit juice for the soy beverage; try orange or cranberry juice or peach or pear nectar.

NUTRITIONAL VALUE
per serving

Calories	127
Fat, total	2 g
Fat, saturated	0 g
Cholesterol	0 mg
Sodium	31 mg
Carbohydrate	26 g
Fiber	2 g
Protein	2 g
Calcium	84 mg
Iron	1 mg

Mango Smoothie

Makes 2 servings

Perfect in the morning, as a lunch beverage or as a welcome afternoon pick-me-up, this smoothie is a meal in a glass and a great way to increase your fruit servings for the day!

Tip

For information about preparing mangoes, see page 247.

¾ cup	Lime Sorbet (see recipe, page 287) or GF store-bought lime sorbet	175 mL
¾ cup	fortified soy beverage, lactose-free milk or milk	175 mL
1	very ripe mango, peeled, pitted and cut into cubes	1
⅓ cup	frozen orange juice concentrate	75 mL
1	slice candied ginger, chopped	1

1. In a blender or food processor, purée sorbet, soy beverage, mango, orange juice concentrate and ginger until smooth. Serve immediately.

Variations

Substitute ½ cup (125 mL) Mango Purée (page 288) for the fresh mango.

Substitute lactose-free soy frozen dessert for the Lime Sorbet.

Substitute yogurt for the soy beverage.

You can omit the Lime Sorbet altogether.

NUTRITIONAL VALUE
per serving

Calories	319
Fat, total	7 g
Fat, saturated	6 g
Cholesterol	2 mg
Sodium	84 mg
Carbohydrate	63 g
Fiber	3 g
Protein	6 g
Calcium	169 mg
Iron	2 mg

Cream of Tomato and Leek Soup

Makes 6 cups (1.5 L) (½ cup/125 mL per serving)

Here's an updated cream of tomato soup to serve with our Skillet Cornbread (page 136) on a cold winter's day.

Tips

For instructions on cleaning leeks, roasting garlic and peeling tomatoes, see the Technique Glossary, pages 300–302.

Substitute one 28-oz (796 mL) can diced or whole tomatoes, including juice, for the fresh.

2 tbsp	vegetable oil, lactose-free buttery spread or butter	25 mL
3	leeks, white and light green parts only, cut into ½-inch (1 cm) slices	3
1	bulb garlic, roasted	1
1	carrot, chopped	1
1	stalk celery, chopped	1
1 cup	GF vegetable stock	250 mL
3 tbsp	tomato paste	45 mL
3 lbs	Roma (plum) or beefsteak tomatoes, peeled and chopped	1.5 kg
2	bay leaves	2
1 tsp	dried basil	5 mL
½ tsp	salt	2 mL
¼ tsp	freshly ground black pepper	1 mL
1 cup	fortified soy beverage, lactose-free milk or milk	250 mL

1. In a large saucepan, heat oil over low heat. Add leeks, roasted garlic, carrot and celery. Cover and cook, stirring occasionally, for 10 to 12 minutes, or until tender but not brown. Stir in vegetable stock, tomato paste, tomatoes, bay leaves, basil, salt and pepper; bring to a boil over high heat. Reduce heat to medium-low and simmer, uncovered, for 25 to 30 minutes, or until flavors are developed. Discard bay leaves.

2. Working in small batches, transfer soup to a food processor or blender and purée until smooth.

3. Return puréed soup to saucepan and slowly stir in soy beverage; heat over medium heat just until steaming. Do not let boil, or soup may curdle.

Variation

For a chunky tomato and leek soup, omit the puréeing step and substitute one 28-oz (796 mL) can diced tomatoes for the fortified soy beverage.

NUTRITIONAL VALUE per serving	
Calories	139
Fat, total	5 g
Fat, saturated	0 g
Cholesterol	0 mg
Sodium	649 mg
Carbohydrate	20 g
Fiber	4 g
Protein	3 g
Calcium	91 mg
Iron	3 mg

Lentil Soup

Makes 6 cups (1.5 L) (1 cup/250 mL per serving)

Think you don't have time to make homemade soup? This quick-to-prepare, healthy, nutritious soup will surprise you.

Tips

You can either use a homemade GF chicken stock or reconstitute a commercial GF chicken stock powder.

Recipe can be doubled and frozen as individual servings.

For a creamier soup, purée all or part of the soup before adding the chopped ham.

NUTRITIONAL VALUE per serving	
Calories	346
Fat, total	7 g
Fat, saturated	1 g
Cholesterol	26 mg
Sodium	1,682 mg
Carbohydrate	48 g
Fiber	11 g
Protein	22 g
Calcium	137 mg
Iron	4 mg

4 tsp	vegetable oil	20 mL
2 cups	chopped carrots	500 mL
1½ cups	chopped celery	375 mL
1½ cups	chopped onion	375 mL
6 cups	GF chicken stock or vegetable stock	1.5 L
1	ham bone	1
1 cup	dried red lentils, rinsed	250 mL
1	bay leaf	1
¼ tsp	dried marjoram	1 mL
¼ tsp	freshly ground black pepper	1 mL
1 cup	diced cooked ham	250 mL

1. In a large saucepan, heat oil over low heat. Add carrots, celery and onion. Cover and cook, stirring occasionally, for 5 to 8 minutes, or until tender but not brown. Stir in chicken stock, ham bone, lentils, bay leaf, marjoram and pepper; bring to a boil. Reduce heat to medium-low and simmer, uncovered, for 25 to 30 minutes, or until lentils are tender. Discard bay leaf. Stir in ham and heat through, about 5 minutes.

Variations

Substitute split peas or green lentils for the red lentils and increase the cooking time to 45 to 60 minutes, or until tender.

If you don't have a ham bone, double the amount of marjoram and increase the amount of chicken stock powder or add salt to taste. Or use a plain or smoked pork hock, omit the cooked ham and add chopped meat from the pork hock.

Spinach and Pear Soup

Makes 6 cups (1.5 L) (1 cup/250 mL) per serving)

This refreshingly flavorful soup can be served hot or cold.

Tips

The first step cooks very slowly to develop a good flavor base.

We recommend rinsing the spinach under cold running water, even though it is labeled as washed.

2 tsp	extra-virgin olive oil	10 mL
3	pears, peeled and chopped	3
2	cloves garlic, minced	2
2	potatoes, peeled and diced	2
1	onion, chopped	1
2 cups	GF chicken stock or vegetable stock	500 mL
6 oz	fresh baby spinach (about 6 cups/1.5 L)	175 g
1 tbsp	Dijon mustard	15 mL
¼ tsp	ground nutmeg	1 mL
1 tsp	freshly squeezed lemon juice	5 mL
	Salt and freshly ground white pepper	

1. In a large saucepan, heat oil over low heat. Add pears, garlic, potatoes and onion; cover and cook, stirring occasionally, for about 20 minutes, or until tender but not brown. Add stock and bring to a boil over medium-high heat. Reduce heat to low and simmer, uncovered, for 10 minutes, or until potato is tender. Stir in spinach, mustard, nutmeg and lemon juice until spinach is wilted.

2. Working in small batches, transfer soup to a food processor or blender and purée until smooth.

3. Return puréed soup to saucepan and heat over medium heat just until steaming. Season to taste with salt and pepper. Serve hot or, to serve cold, cover and refrigerate for at least 1 hour, until chilled. Store in the refrigerator for up to 3 days.

Variation

Substitute chopped Swiss chard, strawberry Swiss chard or kale for the spinach.

NUTRITIONAL VALUE per serving	
Calories	93
Fat, total	2 g
Fat, saturated	0 g
Cholesterol	0 mg
Sodium	327 mg
Carbohydrate	18 g
Fiber	3 g
Protein	3 g
Calcium	44 mg
Iron	1 mg

Gazpacho

Makes 4½ cups (1.050 L) (¾ cup/175 mL per serving)

This traditional cold soup from southern Spain smells like a fresh summer salad.

Tip

In the summer, we like to triple this recipe and keep it in the refrigerator, ready for lunch.

1½ cups	tomato juice	375 mL
3	large tomatoes, peeled, seeded and diced	3
2	stalks celery, diced	2
2	green onions, sliced	2
2	cloves garlic, minced	2
½	English cucumber, diced	½
½	red bell pepper, diced	½
¼ cup	snipped fresh parsley	50 mL
2 tbsp	red wine vinegar	25 mL
2 tbsp	extra-virgin olive oil	25 mL
¼ tsp	salt	1 mL
¼ tsp	GF Worcestershire sauce	1 mL

1. In a large glass bowl, combine tomato juice, tomatoes, celery, green onions, garlic, cucumber, bell pepper, parsley, vinegar, oil, salt and Worcestershire sauce. Cover and refrigerate for at least 2 hours, until chilled. Store in the refrigerator for up to 3 days.

Variation

Substitute tomato-vegetable juice for the tomato juice.

NUTRITIONAL VALUE per serving	
Calories	81
Fat, total	5 g
Fat, saturated	1 g
Cholesterol	0 mg
Sodium	266 mg
Carbohydrate	8 g
Fiber	2 g
Protein	2 g
Calcium	39 mg
Iron	1 mg

Snow Pea and Red Pepper Salad

Makes 4 servings

This salad is pretty as a picture — colorful, crisp and delicious!

Tips

For info on mesclun, see the Ingredient Glossary, page 296.

Mushrooms can be stored in a paper bag in the refrigerator for up to 4 days.

For information on toasting seeds, see the Technique Glossary, page 301.

Remove the tough string from the snow peas by grasping the stem end and pulling.

Sesame Orange Dressing

⅓ cup	freshly squeezed orange juice	75 mL
2 tbsp	extra-virgin olive oil	25 mL
2 tbsp	white wine vinegar	25 mL
2 tbsp	sesame seeds, toasted	25 mL
1	clove garlic, minced	1
1 tsp	granulated sugar	5 mL
Pinch	salt	Pinch

Salad

1	package (10 oz/300 g) mesclun	1
6 oz	snow peas	175 g
1	red bell pepper, cut into ¼-inch (0.5 cm) strips	1
4 oz	mushrooms, sliced	125 g

1. *Prepare the dressing:* In a small bowl, whisk together orange juice, oil, vinegar, sesame seeds, garlic, sugar and salt. Set aside for at least 1 hour. Store in a covered jar in the refrigerator for up to 3 weeks.

2. *Prepare the salad:* Using four individual salad plates, divide the mesclun evenly. Top each with one-quarter of the snow peas, red peppers and mushrooms. Serve drizzled with dressing.

Variations

Substitute walnut oil for the olive oil.

If you prefer softer snow peas, blanch them for 1 to 2 minutes.

NUTRITIONAL VALUE per serving

Calories	149
Fat, total	9 g
Fat, saturated	1 g
Cholesterol	0 mg
Sodium	97 mg
Carbohydrate	14 g
Fiber	4 g
Protein	4 g
Calcium	73 mg
Iron	3 mg

Quinoa Salsa Salad

Salsa spices up an easy dressing for this make-ahead salad.

Tips

See the Technique Glossary, page 301, for information on cooking quinoa and "Cooking Rice" on page 46 for information on cooking wild rice.

Use leftover black beans, kidney beans and corn in chili, bean salad or salsa.

Dressing

3 tbsp	GF salsa	45 mL
1 tbsp	extra-virgin olive oil	15 mL
2 tsp	cider vinegar	10 mL
2 tsp	chili powder	10 mL
	Salt and freshly ground black pepper	

Salad

1 cup	cooked quinoa	250 mL
1 cup	cooked wild rice	250 mL
½ cup	rinsed, drained canned black beans	125 mL
½ cup	rinsed, drained canned red kidney beans	125 mL
½ cup	· corn kernels	125 mL
½ cup	chopped celery	125 mL
½ cup	chopped red bell pepper	125 mL
¼ cup	chopped red onion	50 mL
2 tbsp	snipped fresh cilantro	25 mL

1. *Prepare the dressing:* In a small bowl, whisk together salsa, oil, vinegar, chili powder and salt and pepper to taste. Set aside for at least 1 hour. Store in a covered jar in the refrigerator for up to 3 weeks.

2. *Prepare the salad:* In a large bowl, combine quinoa, wild rice, black beans, kidney beans, corn, celery, red pepper, red onion and cilantro.

3. Pour dressing over salad and toss well to coat. Cover and refrigerate for at least 4 hours or overnight to allow flavors to develop and blend.

Variation

Substitute long-grain brown or white rice for the wild rice.

NUTRITIONAL VALUE
per serving

Calories	103
Fat, total	2 g
Fat, saturated	0 g
Cholesterol	0 mg
Sodium	96 mg
Carbohydrate	18 g
Fiber	3 g
Protein	4 g
Calcium	20 mg
Iron	1 mg

Six-Bean Tomato Salad

Makes 4 servings

We enjoy this bean medley because it provides a good variety of taste when you're preparing only a small amount.

Tips

Beans are a source of iron and calcium, as well as a very high source of fiber, while still being low in fat.

The bean medley we used had chickpeas (garbanzos), red kidney beans, black-eyed peas, white kidney beans, romano beans and baby lima beans.

1	can (19 oz/540 mL) six-bean medley, rinsed and drained	1
⅓ cup	Roasted Garlic Dressing (see recipe, page 83), divided	75 mL
1 cup	cherry tomatoes, halved	250 mL
½	head romaine lettuce, torn in pieces	½

1. In a large bowl, combine beans and ¼ cup (50 mL) of the Roasted Garlic Dressing, tossing to coat. Cover and refrigerate for at least 4 hours or for up to 1 day.

2. Add tomatoes and romaine to bowl. Toss with the remaining dressing.

Variations

Add ½ cup (125 mL) 1-inch (2.5 cm) pieces cooked green beans.

To make salad for a large crowd, use 1 can (19 oz/ 540 mL) of each of four different beans — white kidney, red kidney, pinto, black, chickpea (garbanzo) or large lentils. Multiply other ingredient quantities by four.

Substitute whole grape tomatoes for the cherry tomatoes.

NUTRITIONAL VALUE
per serving

Calories	126
Fat, total	10 g
Fat, saturated	1 g
Cholesterol	0 mg
Sodium	226 mg
Carbohydrate	7 g
Fiber	2 g
Protein	2 g
Calcium	17 mg
Iron	1 mg

Crab and Melon Salad

Makes 4 servings

On those hot, humid summer days, nothing is more refreshing that this luncheon salad.

Tips

For instructions on cooking quinoa, see the Technique Glossary, page 301.

♦

You can use thawed frozen or drained canned crabmeat. Just make sure, when purchasing crabmeat, to check the ingredients label for wheat starch; it is sometimes added in processing. One 10 oz (300 g) package of frozen crabmeat yields 1¾ cups (425 mL) chopped.

♦

Remember to wash the outside of the cantaloupe before peeling.

1¾ cups	GF crabmeat, chopped	425 mL
2 tbsp	freshly squeezed lemon juice	25 mL
1 cup	cooked quinoa, chilled	250 mL
2	stalks celery, diced	2
½	small cantaloupe, peeled, seeded and chopped	½
¼ cup	GF lactose-free mayonnaise or GF mayonnaise	50 mL
¼ cup	GF lactose-free sour cream or GF sour cream	50 mL
	Salt and freshly ground white pepper	
4 cups	torn mixed greens	1 L

1. In a large bowl, combine crabmeat and lemon juice. Stir in quinoa, celery and cantaloupe.

2. In a small bowl, combine mayonnaise and sour cream. Add to crab mixture and combine gently with a fork. Season to taste with salt and pepper. Serve immediately or cover and refrigerate for up to 2 days. Spoon on top of greens just before serving.

Variations

Substitute cooked brown rice for half of the quinoa and honeydew melon for the cantaloupe.

Substitute lactose-free plain yogurt for the sour cream.

NUTRITIONAL VALUE per serving

Calories	297
Fat, total	16 g
Fat, saturated	2 g
Cholesterol	73 mg
Sodium	461 mg
Carbohydrate	18 g
Fiber	3 g
Protein	21 g
Calcium	99 mg
Iron	2 mg

Danish Potato Salad

Here's a lighter version of a classic summer salad!

Tip

Select the smallest potatoes of the same size or cut larger potatoes into bite-size pieces. Low-starch and new potatoes will keep their shape when simmered. There's no need to peel — the red skin adds both color and fiber.

1½ lbs	new red-skinned potatoes	750 g
6	slices GF bacon, cooked crisp and crumbled	6

Dressing

2 tsp	extra-virgin olive oil	10 mL
1	small onion, finely chopped	1
1 tbsp	amaranth flour	15 mL
¾ cup	GF chicken or vegetable stock	175 mL
3 tbsp	freshly squeezed lemon juice	45 mL
1 tbsp	Dijon mustard	15 mL
1 tbsp	liquid honey	15 mL
½ tsp	celery seeds	2 mL
Pinch	freshly ground black pepper	Pinch

1. In a large pot, cover potatoes with cold water; bring to a boil over high heat. Salt water, reduce heat to medium-low and simmer for 15 to 20 minutes, or until potatoes are fork-tender. Drain and transfer to a large bowl; keep warm.

2. *Meanwhile, prepare the dressing:* In a large skillet, heat oil over medium heat. Add onion and cook, stirring, for 2 to 3 minutes, or until tender. Stir in amaranth flour and cook, stirring, for 1 to 2 minutes, or until mixture has the appearance of dry sand. Whisk in stock, lemon juice, mustard, honey, celery seeds and pepper; bring to a boil. Reduce heat to medium-low and simmer, stirring occasionally, for 5 to 7 minutes, or until slightly thickened.

3. Pour hot dressing over potatoes in bowl and add bacon. Stir gently until evenly coated. Serve hot or, to serve cold, cover and refrigerate for at least 2 hours, until chilled, or for up to 1 day.

NUTRITIONAL VALUE per serving	
Calories	115
Fat, total	3 g
Fat, saturated	1 g
Cholesterol	4 mg
Sodium	200 mg
Carbohydrate	20 g
Fiber	1 g
Protein	3 g
Calcium	13 mg
Iron	0 mg

Variation

For a spicier version of this salad, add a pinch of cayenne pepper or a few drops of GF hot sauce with the pepper.

Pasta Salad

Makes 4 servings

Summertime demands ice-cold salads. You can put this one together in the morning before you leave for work, to enjoy that night for supper.

Tips

Follow package directions for cooking pasta, as instructions vary.

Cook extra GF pasta and keep it in the freezer so it's on hand when you need it. Thaw overnight in the refrigerator, in the microwave or in a pot of boiling water.

1½ cups	Tomato Pasta Sauce (see recipe, page 110)	375 mL
1 cup	small GF rotini, cooked, rinsed in cold water and drained	250 mL
2	stalks celery, cut into ¼-inch (0.5 cm) slices	2
2	green onions, cut into ¼-inch (0.5 cm) slices	2
⅓ cup	diced green bell pepper	75 mL
	Salt and freshly ground white pepper	

1. In a large bowl, combine pasta sauce, pasta, celery, green onions and green pepper. Cover and refrigerate for at least 2 hours to allow flavors to develop and blend. Season to taste with salt and pepper just before serving. Store in the refrigerator for up to 3 days.

Variation

Use a different type of pasta, but make sure to choose a shape that extra sauce clings to, such as elbows or shells.

NUTRITIONAL VALUE per serving	
Calories	155
Fat, total	2 g
Fat, saturated	0 g
Cholesterol	0 mg
Sodium	680 mg
Carbohydrate	25 g
Fiber	3 g
Protein	4 g
Calcium	95 mg
Iron	3 mg

Roasted Garlic Dressing

**Makes ⅔ cup
(150 mL)
(2 tbsp/25 mL
per serving)**

Garlic becomes very sweet with roasting and adds a subtle flavor to this dressing. It's perfect for Six-Bean Tomato Salad (page 79), a Caesar salad or drizzled over fresh tomatoes and cucumbers.

Tips

For info on roasting garlic, see the Technique Glossary, page 300.

Whisk or shake dressing to combine just before adding to salad.

For better flavor, let dressing stand at room temperature for at least 30 minutes before serving.

1	head garlic, roasted and mashed	1
⅓ cup	extra-virgin olive oil	75 mL
¼ cup	roasted garlic–flavored rice vinegar	50 mL
1 tsp	granulated sugar	5 mL
½ tsp	salt	2 mL
¼ tsp	freshly ground white pepper	1 mL

1. In a small bowl, whisk together garlic, oil, vinegar, sugar, salt and pepper. Cover and refrigerate overnight to allow flavors to develop and blend. Store in a covered jar in the refrigerator for up to 3 weeks.

Variations

Substitute white wine vinegar for the flavored rice vinegar.

Use any flavor of purchased rice vinegar, such as basil and oregano or red pepper.

NUTRITIONAL VALUE per serving	
Calories	120
Fat, total	13 g
Fat, saturated	2 g
Cholesterol	0 mg
Sodium	194 mg
Carbohydrate	2 g
Fiber	0 g
Protein	0 g
Calcium	6 mg
Iron	0 mg

Gluten Cross-Contamination in the Kitchen

"Cross-contamination" is the transfer of biological, chemical or physical contaminants to food while processing, preparing, cooking or serving it. Such transfers usually occur when people handle the food. Bacterial cross-contamination can occur when you handle raw then cooked meats, or cut raw meats then vegetables on the same board with the same knife.

If your kitchen is not completely gluten-free, here are a few extra points to help you avoid cross-contamination:

1. Remember, crumbs can hide in silverware and utensil drawers, as well as in baking dishes and cooling racks.

   ◆

2. Keep a separate cupboard and work area for GF baking supplies and utensils.

   ◆

3. Purchase a toaster, frying pan, colander, spatula, microwave and bread machine baking pan to use exclusively for GF foods.

   ◆

4. Purchase and label separate peanut butter, jam, cream cheese and butter to prevent wheat crumbs from contaminating them when a non-GF family member dips in.

   ◆

5. Purchase squeeze bottles for mustard, GF mayonnaise, relish and GF barbecue sauce.

   ◆

6. Keep the top shelf in the refrigerator for GF products, so wheat crumbs can't drop in. Be sure to cover all foods in the refrigerator, whether GF or not.

   ◆

7. If you use a knife block, ensure that all knives are washed well and rinsed before storing. Better yet, keep separate knives and cutting boards for exclusive GF use.

   ◆

8. Be extra cautious when using wooden cutting boards, and when serving foods in wooden salad bowls, serving dishes or trays.

   ◆

9. Wipe counters frequently, rinsing and changing cloths between each task to prevent cross-contamination.

The Main Event

Florentine Pizza

Makes 6 servings

This vegetarian Greek-style pizza has generous amounts of spinach, feta cheese and Kalamata olives.

Tips

Drain spinach well in a colander before drying completely with paper towels.

Reheat leftover pizza under the broiler to enjoy crisp pizza.

♦ Preheat oven to 400°F (200°C)

1	package (10 oz/300 g) fresh baby spinach (about 10 cups/2.5 L), washed and trimmed	1
1	partially baked Pizza Crust (see recipe, page 218)	1
2	cloves garlic, minced	2
1/2 cup	grated lactose-free Parmesan cheese or Parmesan cheese	125 mL
1 tbsp	extra-virgin olive oil	15 mL
2 tsp	dried oregano	10 mL
1 cup	lactose-free soy feta or feta cheese, crumbled	250 mL
1/2 cup	Kalamata olives, sliced	125 mL

1. In a microwave-safe bowl, microwave spinach, uncovered, on High for 2 to 3 minutes, stirring halfway through. Drain, place between layers of paper towels and pat dry. Spread over crust in a single layer to within 1/4 inch (0.5 cm) of the edges.

2. In a small bowl, combine garlic, Parmesan cheese, oil and oregano. Spread over spinach; sprinkle with feta cheese and olives.

3. Bake in preheated oven for 20 to 25 minutes, or until spinach is crisp and top is golden. Serve hot.

Variations

For a stronger, more prominent garlic flavor, add an extra 1 to 2 cloves minced garlic.

Add 1/2 cup (125 mL) snipped sun-dried tomatoes.

Substitute Swiss chard or kale for the spinach and microwave until wilted.

NUTRITIONAL VALUE
per serving

Calories	316
Fat, total	15 g
Fat, saturated	6 g
Cholesterol	29 mg
Sodium	863 mg
Carbohydrate	35 g
Fiber	5 g
Protein	13 g
Calcium	300 mg
Iron	4 mg

Sausage and Leek Pizza

This recipe is sure to fill up the hungriest teen.

Tip

For information on cleaning leeks, see the Technique Glossary, page 301.

♦ *Preheat oven to 400°F (200°C)*

1 lb	GF pork sausage, casings removed and meat crumbled	500 g
3	carrots, finely chopped	3
3	leeks, white and light green parts only, cut into ½-inch (1 cm) slices	3
1 cup	sliced mushrooms	250 mL
2 tbsp	crumbled dried rosemary	25 mL
2 tbsp	dry white wine	25 mL
1	partially baked Pizza Crust (see recipe, page 218)	1
1 cup	shredded lactose-free mozzarella cheese or mozzarella cheese	250 mL

1. In a large skillet, over medium heat, brown sausage meat until no pink remains. Using a slotted spoon, remove to a plate and set aside. Drain off all but 1 tbsp (15 mL) fat from the skillet.

2. In the fat remaining in the skillet, over medium heat, cook carrots, leeks, mushrooms and rosemary, stirring, for 15 minutes, or until carrots are tender. Drain off fat. Return browned sausage to skillet with wine. Mix gently and set aside to cool slightly.

3. Spread filling over crust to within ¼ inch (0.5 cm) of the edges. Sprinkle with mozzarella cheese.

4. Bake in preheated oven for 20 to 25 minutes, or until cheese is melted and top is golden. Serve hot.

NUTRITIONAL VALUE
per serving

Calories	386
Fat, total	13 g
Fat, saturated	4 g
Cholesterol	23 mg
Sodium	936 mg
Carbohydrate	47 g
Fiber	6 g
Protein	22 g
Calcium	173 mg
Iron	5 mg

Variations

Add ½ cup (125 mL) snipped sun-dried tomatoes with the mozzarella.

Try a mixture of lactose-free Cheddar and mozzarella cheeses.

Substitute unsweetened apple juice for the wine.

Barbecued Tuscan Toastie

Makes 4 to 5 servings

Try this sandwich, and you'll understand the Tuscan attitude to food: "With love, from the heart."

Tips

Choose 2 to 3 kinds of cold cuts, such as GF prosciutto, GF smoked turkey, GF salami or capicollo, either mild, hot or extra-hot.

Choose a couple of kinds of soy cheese or cheese, such as Swiss, Cheddar, mozzarella, American or roasted garlic–flavored.

If you use an indoor contact grill, there's no need to turn the toastie, as both sides cook at once.

NUTRITIONAL VALUE per serving	
Calories	384
Fat, total	17 g
Fat, saturated	1 g
Cholesterol	25 mg
Sodium	758 mg
Carbohydrate	41 g
Fiber	2 g
Protein	16 g
Calcium	32 mg
Iron	2 mg

◆ *Preheat broiler or preheat barbecue or grill to high*

1	Honey Dijon Toastie (see recipe, page 216)	1
1 tbsp	Dijon mustard	15 mL
2 tbsp	GF lactose-free mayonnaise or GF mayonnaise	25 mL
10 oz	thinly sliced GF cold cuts	300 g
6 oz	sliced soy cheese, lactose-free cheese or cheese	180 g
1 cup	mesclun	250 mL
1 tbsp	extra-virgin olive oil	15 mL

1. Slice toastie in half horizontally. Spread the bottom half with mustard and mayonnaise. Arrange cold cuts, soy cheese and mesclun on bottom half, top with other half and press together. Brush both sides of sandwich with olive oil.

2. Place under preheated broiler or on preheated barbecue or grill. Cook, turning once, until sandwich is browned and crisp and cheese is melted. Cut into 4 or 5 wedges. Serve hot.

Black Bean Chili

Makes 6 servings

How about a bowl of protein-rich chili for dinner tonight? This chili is nutritious, colorful and easy.

Tips

Great garnishes for chili include chopped fresh cilantro, chopped green onions, chopped radishes, shredded lactose-free cheese or cheese and lactose-free sour cream or sour cream.

Stovetop Method: In a large saucepan, over medium heat, cook sausage until browned. Drain off fat. Add all other ingredients and bring to a boil over medium-high heat. Reduce heat to low and simmer gently for 1 to 1½ hours.

NUTRITIONAL VALUE per serving

Calories	173
Fat, total	3 g
Fat, saturated	1 g
Cholesterol	5 mg
Sodium	920 mg
Carbohydrate	28 g
Fiber	7 g
Protein	13 g
Calcium	64 mg
Iron	3 mg

◆ 3½- to 6-quart slow cooker

8 oz	GF hot Italian sausage, cut into ½-inch (1 cm) slices	250 g
2 to 3	cloves garlic, finely chopped	2 to 3
1	green bell pepper, chopped	1
1	onion, chopped	1
1	can (19 oz/540 mL) black beans, rinsed and drained	1
1	can (12 oz/341 mL) corn kernels, drained	1
1 cup	canned chopped tomatoes, with juice	250 mL
½ cup	GF chicken stock	125 mL
1	bay leaf	1
1 tbsp	chili powder	15 mL
1½ tsp	cumin seeds	7 mL
1½ tsp	dried oregano	7 mL
Pinch	cayenne pepper	Pinch
	Salt and freshly ground black pepper	

1. In a skillet, over medium heat, cook sausage until browned. Drain off fat.

2. In slow cooker stoneware, combine sausage, garlic to taste, green pepper, onion, black beans, corn, tomatoes, stock, bay leaf, chili powder, cumin seeds, oregano and cayenne. Cover and cook on High for 2 to 3 hours or on Low for 5 to 6 hours, until hot and bubbling. Remove bay leaf and season to taste with salt and pepper.

Variations

Substitute kidney beans for the black beans.

Vegetarian Chili: Use GF vegetable stock instead of chicken stock and omit the sausage.

Salmon Fillets with Lime Dijon Sauce

Makes 4 servings

To escape to the tropics without leaving home, serve this tasty dish with jasmine rice and pineapple, coconut or mango.

Tips

Leaving the skin on the fillets helps prevent the salmon from breaking up.

In a pinch, the lime sauce can be prepared at the last minute. Only the strength of flavor varies.

Barbecue Method: Grill salmon, brushed with honey-lime mixture, on a preheated barbecue lightly brushed with oil.

NUTRITIONAL VALUE per serving	
Calories	369
Fat, total	17 g
Fat, saturated	5 g
Cholesterol	89 mg
Sodium	491 mg
Carbohydrate	16 g
Fiber	0 g
Protein	36 g
Calcium	34 mg
Iron	2 mg

♦ *Broiler pan, lightly brushed with oil*

Lime Dijon Sauce

1 cup	lactose-free sour cream or sour cream	250 mL
1 tbsp	snipped fresh chives	15 mL
1 tsp	liquid honey	5 mL
1 tsp	Dijon mustard	5 mL
2 tsp	grated lime zest	10 mL

Salmon

2 tbsp	liquid honey	25 mL
1 tbsp	grated lime zest	15 mL
1 tbsp	freshly squeezed lime juice	15 mL
1 tbsp	Dijon mustard	15 mL
4	salmon fillets, 1 inch (2.5 cm) thick (each 6 oz/175 g)	4

1. *Prepare the sauce:* In a small bowl, combine sour cream, chives, honey, mustard and lime zest. Cover and refrigerate for at least 1 hour, to allow flavors to blend, or for up 24 hours. Preheat broiler.

2. *Prepare the salmon:* In a small bowl, combine honey, lime zest, lime juice and mustard. Place salmon on prepared pan and coat both sides evenly with honey-lime mixture.

3. Broil for 5 to 6 minutes per side, turning once, or until fish is opaque and flakes easily when tested with a fork.

4. Serve salmon with cold sauce on the side.

Variations

Substitute any firm fish fillet, such as halibut, tuna or swordfish, for the salmon.

Substitute dill or basil for the chives and lemon zest and juice for the lime.

Scallops Provençal

Savor this modern version of a traditional French dish.

Tips

Fresh scallops should be large and off-white. They should have a sweet, fresh smell and a moist sheen.

Frozen scallops are available in a 13-oz (400 g) package, which contains 20 to 35 scallops. This amount can be used in this recipe. Thaw according to package directions or add frozen and double the cooking time.

4 oz	GF linguine	125 g
1 lb	sea scallops	500 g
3 cups	Tomato Pasta Sauce (see recipe, page 110)	750 mL
⅓ cup	Kalamata olives, pitted and thickly sliced	75 mL
¼ cup	chopped fresh Italian (flat-leaf) parsley	50 mL
	Salt and freshly ground black pepper	

1. Cook pasta according to package directions, or just until tender. Drain well and rinse under cold running water.
2. In a deep saucepan, over medium-low heat, combine pasta, scallops, Tomato Pasta Sauce, olives and parsley. Cover and simmer for 5 minutes, or until scallops are opaque and just firm to the touch. Season to taste with salt and pepper.

Variation
Substitute 2 to 3 lbs (1 to 1.5 kg) of mussels for the scallops. Mussels will cook in about 6 minutes. The shells should open when cooked. Discard any that do not open.

NUTRITIONAL VALUE per serving	
Calories	202
Fat, total	3 g
Fat, saturated	0 g
Cholesterol	38 mg
Sodium	610 mg
Carbohydrate	18 g
Fiber	2 g
Protein	22 g
Calcium	84 mg
Iron	2 mg

Coconut Shrimp

Makes 6 servings

Sweet and crunchy, this popular restaurant appetizer is surprisingly easy to make — and it's great as a main course, too!

Tips

Purchase shrimp either fresh or frozen. Before using, thaw frozen shrimp according to package directions.

This recipe serves 6 as an appetizer.

♦ *Preheat oven to 400°F (200°C)*
♦ *Baking sheet, lightly greased*

2	eggs, lightly beaten	2
1 tbsp	GF mild curry paste	15 mL
1 cup	unsweetened flaked coconut	250 mL
½ cup	almond flour	125 mL
⅓ cup	amaranth flour	75 mL
24	large shrimp (about 1 lb/500 g), with tails left on, peeled and deveined	24
	GF mango chutney or other dipping sauce	

1. In a small bowl, combine eggs and curry paste. In a shallow dish or pie plate, combine coconut and almond flour. Place amaranth flour in another shallow dish.

2. Holding shrimp by their tails, dip into egg mixture, coating generously. Dip into amaranth flour, then back into egg mixture. Dip into coconut mixture, pressing to coat well. Arrange in a single layer on prepared baking sheet. Discard any excess egg mixture, amaranth flour and coconut mixture.

3. Bake in preheated oven for 10 to 12 minutes, or until golden brown. Transfer to a serving plate and serve immediately with mango chutney.

> **To make this recipe egg-free**
> Substitute ½ cup (125 mL) lactose-free plain yogurt or yogurt for the eggs

Variations

If you like finer coconut, use shredded.

Substitute cornstarch for the amaranth flour.

Instead of baking shrimp, place 4 at a time in a deep fryer or saucepan filled with vegetable oil heated to 375°F (190°C); deep-fry for 1 to 2 minutes, or until golden brown.

Cioppino

This Italian fisherman's stew, made with tomatoes and a variety of shellfish, is easy enough for a weeknight dinner, yet impressive enough for a gourmet meal.

Tips

See the Technique Glossary, page 301, for information on cleaning leeks.

There are about 12 sea scallops and 8 to 10 extra-large shrimp or 5 to 7 jumbo shrimp in 8 oz (250 g).

To steam mussels, cook in 1 inch (2.5 cm) of boiling water for 5 minutes. Mussel shells should open when cooked. Discard any that do not open.

NUTRITIONAL VALUE per serving	
Calories	274
Fat, total	4 g
Fat, saturated	1 g
Cholesterol	123 mg
Sodium	837 mg
Carbohydrate	26 g
Fiber	3 g
Protein	32 g
Calcium	170 mg
Iron	7 mg

• 3½- to 6-quart slow cooker

2	leeks, white and light green parts only, cut into 1-inch (2.5 cm) slices	2
2	cloves garlic, minced	2
1	red bell pepper, cut into ¼-inch (0.5 cm) slices	1
1	yellow bell pepper, cut into ¼-inch (0.5 cm) slices	1
1	stalk celery, chopped	1
1	can (28 oz/796 mL) chopped tomatoes, with juice	1
½ cup	GF chicken stock	125 mL
2 tsp	dried basil	10 mL
8 oz	sea scallops	250 g
8 oz	extra-large or jumbo shrimp, cooked and peeled	250 g
16	mussels, steamed	16
¼ cup	dry red wine	50 mL

1. In slow cooker stoneware, combine leeks, garlic, red pepper, yellow pepper, celery, tomatoes, stock and basil. Cover and cook on Low for 6 to 8 hours, or until stew is hot and bubbling and vegetables are tender.
2. Fifteen minutes before serving, turn slow cooker to High; add scallops, shrimp, mussels and red wine. Cover and cook for 15 minutes, or until scallops are opaque.

Variations

When tomatoes are in season, substitute 6 chopped fresh Roma (plum) tomatoes for the canned.

Add 4 oz (125 g) firm-fleshed white fish, or substitute fish for some of the shellfish. Try monkfish, salmon, tilapia or halibut.

Substitute GF vegetable or beef stock for the chicken stock.

Substitute tomato-vegetable juice for the wine.

Paella

Enjoy our rustic Spanish dish of rice, vegetables, meats and seafood seasoned with saffron. You can choose to include any meats and seafood you like — we've called for some of our favorites.

Tips

Sofrito is Spanish for "lightly fried."

As soon as this dish is in the oven, relax and enjoy the company of family or guests — there's no need to stir it.

Mussel and clam shells should open when cooked. Discard any that do not open.

NUTRITIONAL VALUE per serving	
Calories	566
Fat, total	14 g
Fat, saturated	4 g
Cholesterol	107 mg
Sodium	973 mg
Carbohydrate	61 g
Fiber	1 g
Protein	45 g
Calcium	65 mg
Iron	3 mg

♦ *Preheat oven to 400°F (200°C), with rack set in lowest position*
♦ *14-inch (35 cm) paella pan, 2½ inches (6 cm) deep*

Sofrito

2 tsp	extra-virgin olive oil	10 mL
2 oz	cooked ham, diced	60 g
1	onion, diced	1
1	clove garlic, minced	1
1	green bell pepper, diced	1
1	large tomato, chopped	1

Base

8 oz	garlic-smoked pork sausage	250 g
3 cups	long-grain white rice	750 mL
1 tsp	salt	5 mL
¼ tsp	ground saffron	1 mL
6 cups	boiling water	1.5 L
6	medium shrimp, shells on	6
6	hard-shelled clams	6
6	mussels	6
4	skinless boneless chicken breasts, cut in half	4
½ cup	fresh or frozen peas, thawed	125 mL

1. *Prepare the sofrito:* In a skillet, heat olive oil over medium heat. Add ham and cook, stirring, for 2 or 3 minutes, or until browned. Add onion, garlic, green pepper and tomato; cook, stirring constantly, for 8 to 10 minutes, or until most of the liquid has evaporated and mixture is thick enough to hold its shape on a spoon. Set aside.

2. *Prepare the base:* With a fork, prick sausage in several places. Place in a saucepan with enough cold water to cover. Bring to a boil over high heat. Reduce heat to low and simmer gently for 5 minutes, or until no longer pink inside. Drain on paper towels. Slice into ¼-inch (1 cm) thick rounds. Set aside.

Tips

See the Equipment Glossary, page 291, for information on paella pans. If you don't have one, you can use a 14-inch (35 cm) oven-proof skillet — just make sure it is at least 2 inches deep. If you don't have either, use two 8-inch (20 cm) skillets and place half the ingredients in each. The baking time will stay the same.

The sofrito and base can be prepared through Step 2 up to 4 hours ahead. Cover and refrigerate until ready to use.

3. In paella pan, combine sofrito, rice, salt and saffron. Pour in boiling water and return to a boil over high heat, stirring constantly. Remove pan from heat. Arrange shrimp, clams, mussels, chicken and sausage on top of rice and sprinkle dish with peas.

4. Bake, uncovered, in preheated oven for 25 to 30 minutes, or until liquid has been absorbed and rice is tender. Cover loosely with foil or a lint-free towel and let stand for 5 minutes.

Variation

Substitute or add lobster tails to the paella.

Rubbed Roast Chicken

Makes 4 to 6 servings

Tucking a whole chicken into the oven takes just a couple of minutes. Season it for a burst of flavor. This chicken is delicious served hot or cold.

Tips

For more information on thermometers and mezzalunas, see the Equipment Glossary, pages 291–292.

Barbecue method:
Roast on the barbecue for 45 to 50 minutes, using medium heat and the indirect method (see the Technique Glossary, page 299).

NUTRITIONAL VALUE per serving	
Calories	176
Fat, total	8 g
Fat, saturated	2 g
Cholesterol	72 mg
Sodium	70 mg
Carbohydrate	0 g
Fiber	0 g
Protein	24 g
Calcium	18 mg
Iron	1 mg

♦ *Preheat oven to 375°F (190°C)*
♦ *Roasting pan with rack, lightly greased*

1	3- to 3½-lb (1.5 to 2 kg) whole roaster/fryer chicken	1
1 tbsp	extra-virgin olive oil	15 mL
2 tbsp	fresh rosemary	25 mL
1 tbsp	chopped or snipped fresh sage	15 mL
1 tbsp	fresh savory	15 mL
½ tsp	freshly cracked black peppercorns	2 mL
¼ tsp	celery seeds	1 mL

1. Remove neck and giblets from body of chicken. Rinse chicken inside and out with cold water. Pat dry with paper towels. Brush skin with olive oil.

2. Using a mezzaluna or a sharp chef's knife, finely chop rosemary, sage and savory.

3. In a small bowl, combine finely chopped herbs, cracked peppercorns and celery seeds. Sprinkle half of this mixture inside chicken cavity. Using your fingers and starting at the neck end, gently loosen skin from each breast to thigh to form a pocket; rub remaining herb mixture under skin. Tuck wings under back and tie legs together with string. Place on rack in roasting pan.

4. Roast, uncovered, in preheated oven for 1 to 1½ hours, or until a meat thermometer inserted into the thickest part of a thigh registers 185°F (85°C) and juices run clear.

5. Transfer chicken to a platter. Loosely tent with foil and let rest for 5 to 10 minutes before carving.

Variations

In a hurry? Cut whole chicken along the backbone and flatten. Place on broiler pan and roast for 45 to 60 minutes.

Use this tasty rub on chicken pieces or Cornish game hens.

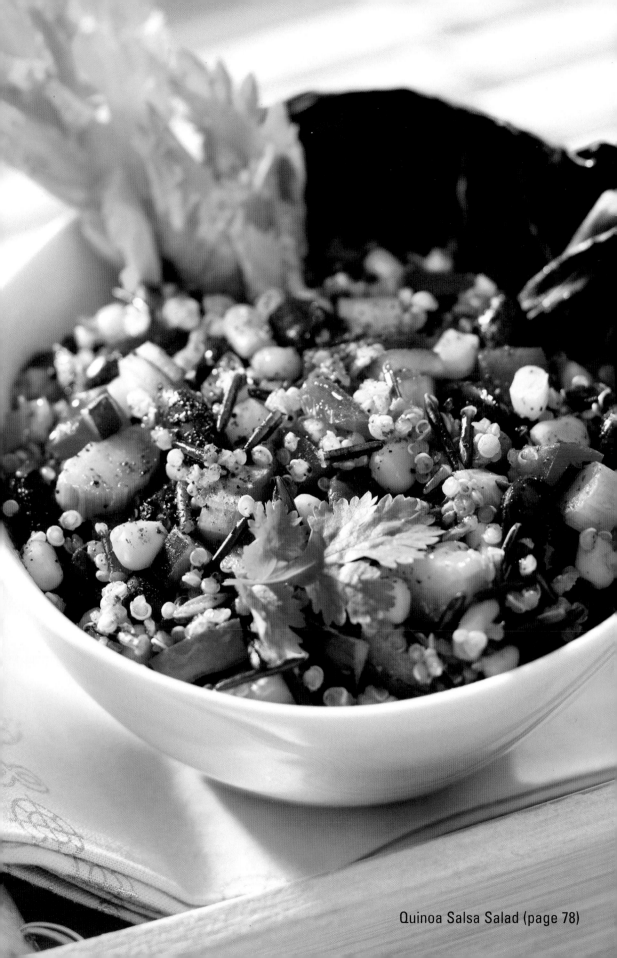

Quinoa Salsa Salad (page 78)

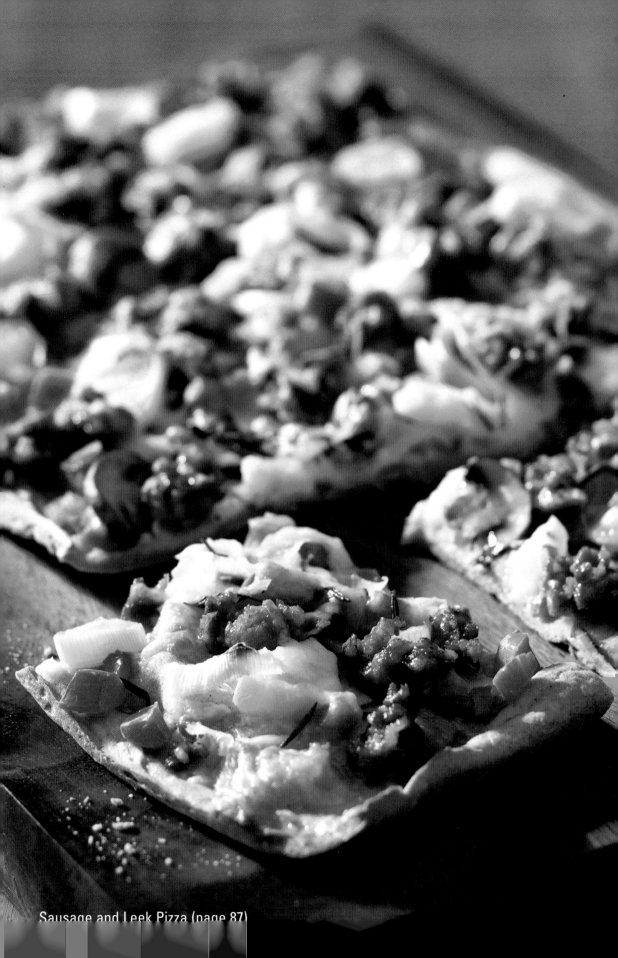

Sausage and Leek Pizza (page 87)

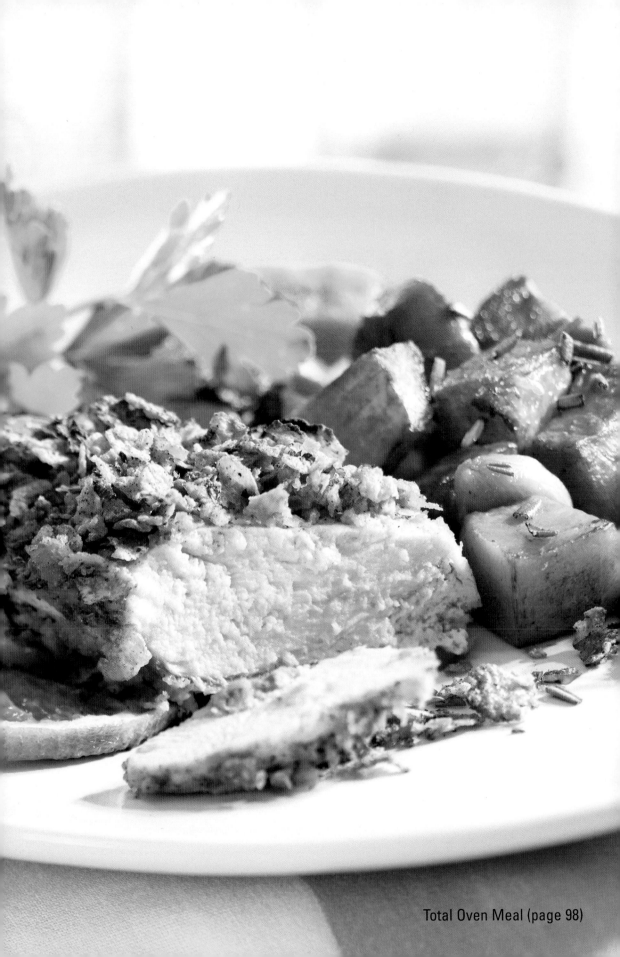

Total Oven Meal (page 98)

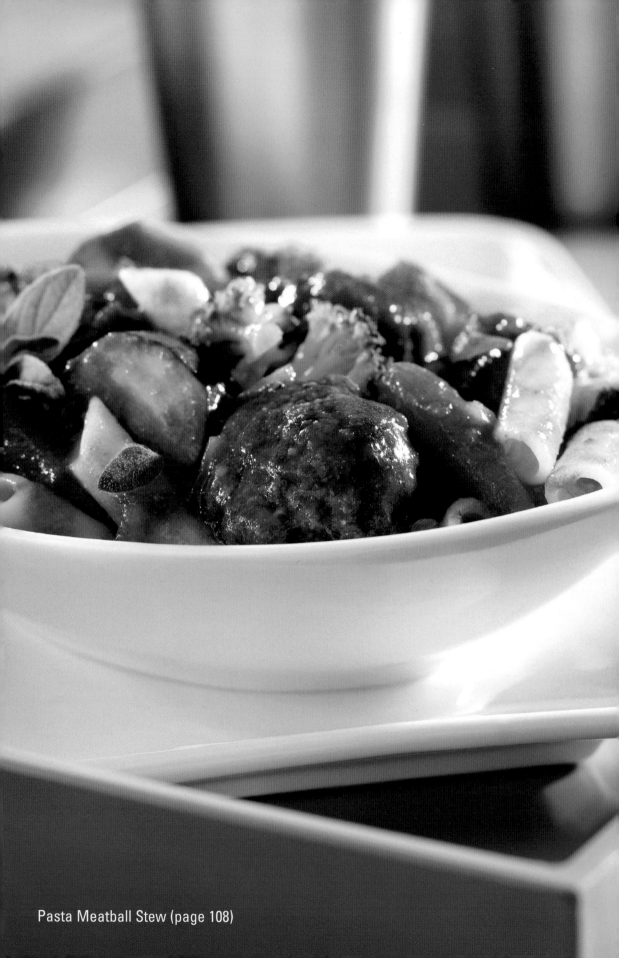

Pasta Meatball Stew (page 108)

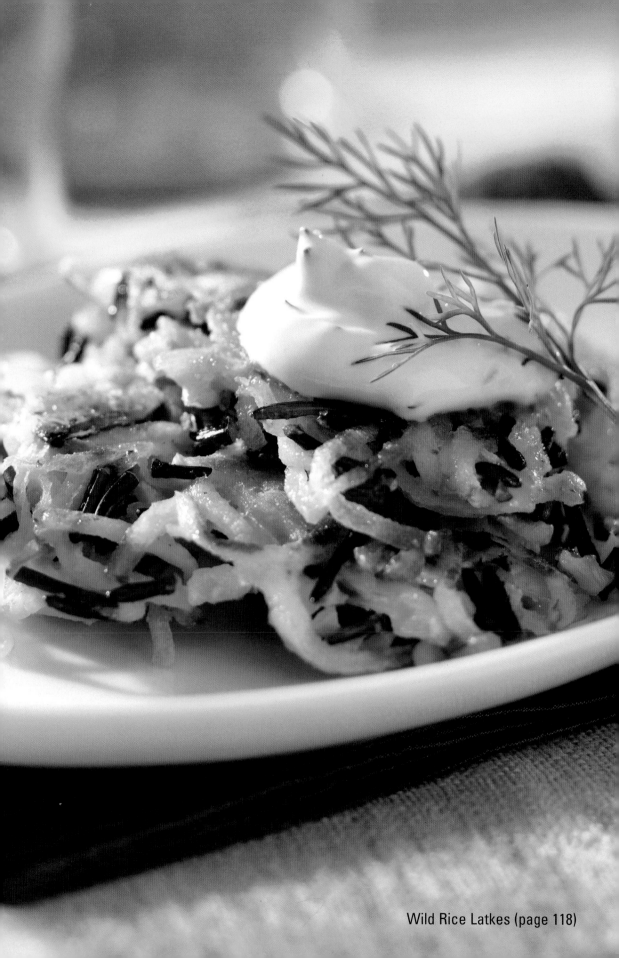

Wild Rice Latkes (page 118)

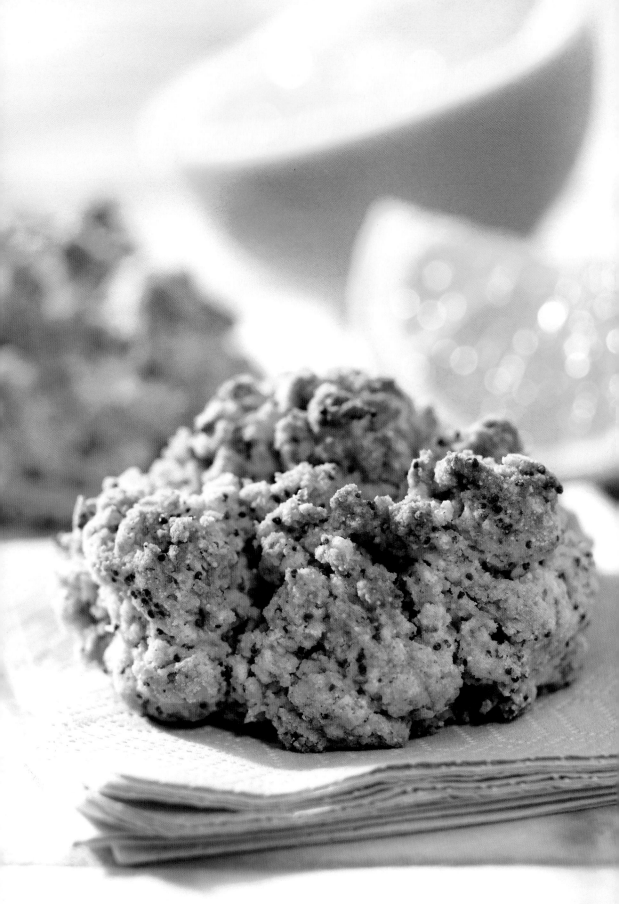

Orange Poppy Seed Biscuits (page 133)

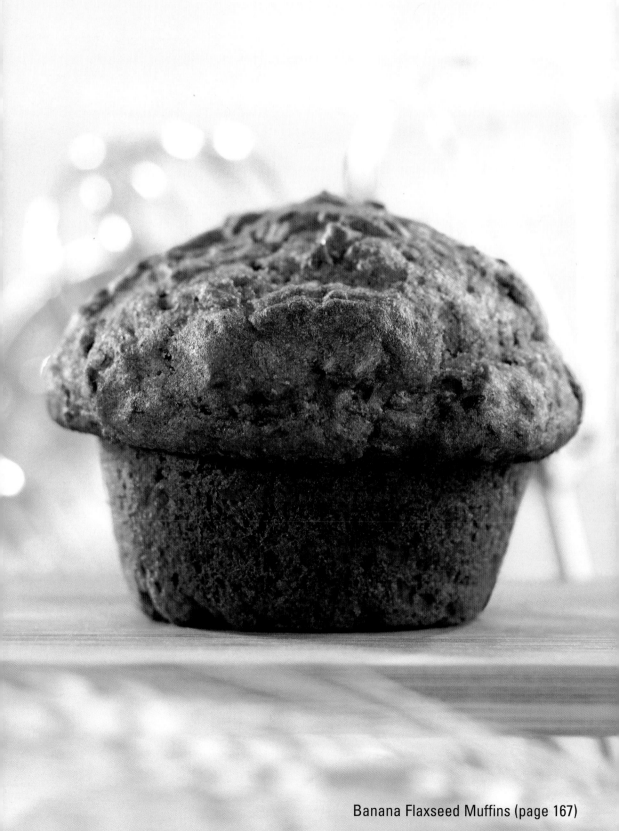

Banana Flaxseed Muffins (page 167)

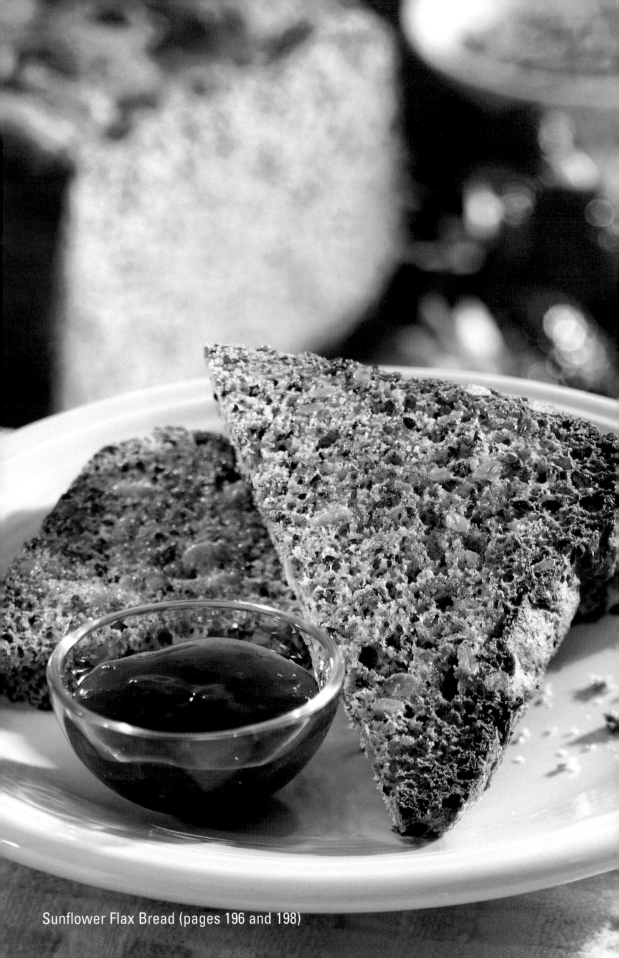
Sunflower Flax Bread (pages 196 and 198)

Asian Chicken Stir-Fry

Makes 2 servings

With our health-conscious, hurry-up lifestyle, stir-fries have become a necessity! We hope you enjoy this one.

Tips

When cutting chicken, cut any longer slices in half to keep pieces even.

Don't try to keep the vegetables warm — covering gives them a steamed, overcooked texture.

◆ 9- to 10-inch (23 to 25 cm) nonstick skillet, 2 inches (5 cm) deep

2	skinless boneless chicken breasts, cut into ¾-inch (2 cm) slices	2
2	cloves garlic, minced	2
½ cup	Mock Soy Sauce (see recipe, page 126) or GF soy sauce	125 mL
2 tsp	vegetable oil	10 mL
12	snow peas, trimmed	12
4	mushrooms, cut in quarters	4
½	red bell pepper, cut into ½-inch (1 cm) slices	½
½	onion, halved lengthwise and thickly sliced	½
1 tbsp	arrowroot starch or cornstarch	15 mL
	Cooked brown rice	

1. In a bowl, combine chicken, garlic and Mock Soy Sauce. Set aside.

2. In a large nonstick skillet, heat oil over medium heat. Add snow peas, mushrooms, red pepper and onion; cook, stirring frequently, for 5 to 7 minutes, or until tender-crisp. Transfer vegetables to a bowl.

3. Drain chicken, reserving soy marinade. Add chicken to the skillet; cook, stirring, for 5 to 8 minutes, or until no longer pink inside. Return vegetables to skillet.

4. In a small bowl, combine arrowroot starch and reserved soy marinade; add to skillet and cook, stirring, for 2 to 3 minutes, or until thickened. Serve over hot rice.

NUTRITIONAL VALUE
per serving

Calories	406
Fat, total	11 g
Fat, saturated	2 g
Cholesterol	137 mg
Sodium	183 mg
Carbohydrate	18 g
Fiber	2 g
Protein	57 g
Calcium	67 mg
Iron	3 mg

Variations

Substitute broccoli florets, sliced celery, julienned carrots, leeks or asparagus for the vegetables.

To save on prep time, purchase a packaged stir-fry mix of fresh vegetables.

For a more Asian flavor, add 1 tsp (5 mL) minced gingerroot to the soy sauce.

Total Oven Meal

Start by preparing the Roasted Vegetables and place in the oven to begin roasting while you prepare the Crunchy Citrus Chicken. Once the chicken's in, there's time to relax with your family or friends before dinner.

Tips

We prefer to use a digital instant-read thermometer (see the Technique Glossary, page 299) to make sure the chicken is cooked.

Discard the plastic bag used for the coating mix — it is not safe to reuse anything when raw chicken is involved.

Crunchy Citrus Chicken

♦ *Preheat oven to 400°F (200°C)*
♦ *13- by 9-inch (3 L) baking pan, lined with foil, lightly greased*

1	lemon	1
1	lime	1
1	orange	1
3 cups	GF corn flakes cereal, coarsely crushed	750 mL
3 tbsp	chopped fresh rosemary	45 mL
2 tbsp	minced fresh parsley	25 mL
2 tsp	paprika	10 mL
½ tsp	salt	2 mL
¼ tsp	freshly ground black pepper	1 mL
4	skinless boneless chicken breasts	4

1. Zest the lemon, lime and orange. Juice half of each citrus fruit. Thinly slice the remaining half of each citrus fruit. Arrange fruit slices in bottom of prepared pan. Set aside.

2. On a pie plate, combine citrus juices. In a plastic bag, combine citrus zests, cereal, rosemary, parsley, paprika, salt and pepper. Roll chicken in citrus juice, then shake in seasoned crumbs. Place on citrus slices and sprinkle with leftover crumb mixture. Discard any excess juice.

3. Bake in preheated oven for 30 to 35 minutes, or until coating is golden brown and crispy, a meat thermometer inserted into the thickest part of a breast registers 170°F (75°C) and chicken is no longer pink inside.

Variation

Substitute fresh Sunflower Flax Bread crumbs (page 196 or 198) for the corn flake crumbs. For instructions on making fresh bread crumbs, see the Technique Glossary, page 299.

NUTRITIONAL VALUE
per serving

Calories	394
Fat, total	2 g
Fat, saturated	1 g
Cholesterol	68 mg
Sodium	820 mg
Carbohydrate	67 g
Fiber	5 g
Protein	33 g
Calcium	56 mg
Iron	12 mg

Looking for a mid-winter vegetable dish? We have fond childhood memories of roasted vegetables served with a Sunday roast.

Tips

If using large parsnips, remove the woody center core.

As rutabaga takes longer to cook, it needs to be cut into slightly smaller cubes than other vegetables.

Turnips and rutabaga can be used interchangeably.

Roasted Vegetables

♦ *Preheat oven to 400°F (200°C)*
♦ *Roasting pan, lightly greased*

3	medium carrots	3
2	large parsnips	2
1	garlic bulb, separated into cloves	1
½	medium rutabaga	½
¼	medium butternut squash	¼
⅓ cup	balsamic vinegar	75 mL
2 tsp	vegetable oil	10 mL
½ tsp	salt	2 mL
¼ tsp	freshly ground black pepper	1 mL
2 tbsp	fresh rosemary	25 mL

1. Peel carrots, parsnips, garlic, rutabaga and squash. Chop carrots, parsnips and squash into 1-inch (2.5 cm) cubes. Chop rutabaga into ¾-inch (2 cm) cubes.

2. In a large bowl, combine vinegar, oil, salt and pepper. Add garlic and chopped vegetables and toss well to coat. Spread in a single layer in prepared pan and cover with foil.

3. Roast in preheated oven for 30 minutes. Remove foil, stir vegetables and sprinkle with rosemary. Roast, uncovered, for 25 to 35 minutes, or until fork-tender.

NUTRITIONAL VALUE per serving	
Calories	113
Fat, total	3 g
Fat, saturated	0 g
Cholesterol	0 mg
Sodium	332 mg
Carbohydrate	21 g
Fiber	4 g
Protein	2 g
Calcium	58 mg
Iron	1 mg

Variations

Substitute red or golden beets for one of the other vegetables.

If you like a sweeter vegetable dish, add 2 tbsp (25 mL) pure maple syrup with the vinegar.

You can add white potatoes or sweet potatoes, or both, for an extra serving of vegetables.

Chicken en Papillote

These chicken packets are impressive yet easy, and you can assemble them ahead. Relax and enjoy your guests, and just pop the envelopes into the oven at a convenient time. Split the envelopes open at the table and let your guests enjoy the fragrance of the cooked food.

Tip

Packets can be prepared through the end of Step 2 and refrigerated for up to 4 hours.

NUTRITIONAL VALUE per serving

Calories	445
Fat, total	16 g
Fat, saturated	4 g
Cholesterol	78 mg
Sodium	522 mg
Carbohydrate	38 g
Fiber	4 g
Protein	37 g
Calcium	279 mg
Iron	3 mg

♦ *Preheat oven to 400°F (200°C)*
♦ *Baking sheet*

16	leaves fresh spinach, washed and trimmed	16
2 cups	cooked jasmine rice (cooked in GF vegetable or chicken stock)	500 mL
½ cup	GF lactose-free pesto	125 mL
4	skinless boneless chicken breasts	4
1	red bell pepper, julienned	1
1	small zucchini, julienned	1
1	carrot, julienned	1
1	leek, white and light green parts only, julienned	1
1	stalk celery, julienned	1

1. Cut four 16- by 15-inch (40 by 37 cm) rectangles of parchment paper. Fold each rectangle in half and cut out the shape of one-half of a heart, with center fold as the center of the heart, covering as much of the paper as possible. When you open up the parchment paper, you'll have a heart-shaped piece.

2. On each open piece of parchment paper, lay one-quarter of the spinach a little off-center on one side of the heart. Top with ½ cup (125 mL) rice and 2 tbsp (25 mL) pesto. Center a chicken breast on top of the pesto, then add one-quarter of the julienned vegetables. Fold one edge of the parchment paper over to meet the other edge, enclosing filling. Seal the packet by making small folds, starting at the top, all around the outer edge of the paper, twisting the paper at the end. Place on baking sheet. Repeat with the remaining parchment paper and ingredients.

Tip
Open packets carefully when testing for doneness, as steam will escape. To avoid being burnt, do not unseal along the outer edge; instead, cut an "X" in the center.

3. Bake in preheated oven for 20 to 25 minutes, or until parchment puffs up with steam, a meat thermometer inserted into a chicken breast registers 170°F (75°C) and chicken is no longer pink inside.

Variations

Substitute freshly squeezed lemon juice or dry white wine for the pesto.

Use aluminum foil in place of the parchment.

Make packets using the full rectangle. Place ingredients in the center, then seal packets by making a drugstore fold (see the Technique Glossary, page 300).

Substitute ½ fennel bulb, 1 cup (250 mL) broccoli florets or 12 snow peas for any of the vegetables.

To Julienne Vegetables

Using a sharp knife, cut vegetables to resemble matchsticks. They should be about ⅛ inch (3 mm) wide, ⅛ inch (3 mm) thick and 2 inches (5 cm) long. Julienned vegetables cook quickly.

Curried Beef with Rice Noodles

Mild or hot — in this dish, you decide how much heat you like. Serve with cucumber slices, orange wedges and pappadams, either mild or spicy, on the side.

Tips

For a more tender flank steak, thinly slice across the grain. Slice while the beef is partially frozen — it's easier.

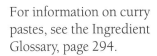

For information on curry pastes, see the Ingredient Glossary, page 294.

1	bunch broccoli (about 1 lb/500 g)	1
10 oz	rice noodles	300 g
2 tsp	vegetable oil	10 mL
1	red onion, thinly sliced	1
3 tbsp	GF mild or hot curry paste	45 mL
¼ tsp	salt	1 mL
1 lb	flank steak, thinly sliced	500 g
3	large tomatoes, cut into wedges	3

1. Cut broccoli into florets. (Reserve stalks for another use or discard.) In a large saucepan of boiling water, blanch for about 3 minutes, or until tender-crisp. Immediately drain and chill under cold running water. Drain and set aside.

2. Meanwhile, in a large bowl, completely cover noodles with boiling water. Let soak for 7 minutes, until softened. Drain and rinse under cold water; set aside.

3. In a large skillet, heat oil over medium-high heat. Cook onion, stirring frequently, for 5 to 8 minutes, or until golden. Using a slotted spoon, remove from pan and set aside.

4. Add curry paste and salt to skillet; cook, stirring, for 30 seconds, or until fragrant. Add steak, in batches, and cook, stirring, for 1 to 2 minutes, or just until rare.

5. Return all beef to pan and add onion, noodles, broccoli and tomatoes. Bring to a boil and heat, stirring gently, for 2 to 3 minutes, or until hot.

Variation

Squeeze fresh lime juice over the noodles.

NUTRITIONAL VALUE
per serving

Calories	540
Fat, total	13 g
Fat, saturated	4 g
Cholesterol	46 mg
Sodium	681 mg
Carbohydrate	74 g
Fiber	7 g
Protein	32 g
Calcium	83 mg
Iron	4 mg

Hawaiian Pineapple Pork

Makes 8 servings

Add a touch of Hawaii to everyday roast pork. Enjoy with coconut rice and fresh baby carrots or green beans.

Tip

If necessary, add ½ cup (125 mL) water to pan while pork is roasting; the liquid tends to evaporate.

♦ *Preheat oven to 400°F (200°C)*
♦ *Roasting pan with rack*

1	fresh pineapple	1
1	bulb garlic, separated into cloves and peeled	1
1 cup	snipped fresh cilantro	250 mL
¼ cup	packed brown sugar	50 mL
2 tbsp	rice vinegar	25 mL
2 tbsp	Mock Soy Sauce (see recipe, page 126) or GF soy sauce	25 mL
1 tsp	cumin seeds	5 mL
1	3-lb (1.5 kg) boneless pork loin roast	1

1. Cut rind from pineapple in wide strips; reserve rind. Core and cut pineapple into bite-size pieces; set aside.

2. In a food processor fitted with a metal blade, process garlic, cilantro, brown sugar, vinegar, Mock Soy Sauce and cumin until smooth.

3. Place pork in roasting pan and coat evenly with spice mixture. Lay pineapple rind (rind side up) over top. Pour 1 cup (250 mL) water into pan.

4. Roast in preheated oven for 45 minutes. Remove rind. Roast, basting every 10 minutes with pan juices, for 10 to 20 minutes, or until a meat thermometer inserted in the center registers 160°F (71°C).

5. Transfer roast to a platter, tent loosely with foil and let stand for 15 to 20 minutes before carving.

6. Meanwhile, add pineapple to roasting pan and roast for 15 to 20 minutes, or until pineapple is warmed through. Serve over roast.

Variation

Use four 10 oz (300 g) pork tenderloins instead of the loin roast. Adjust the cooking time for the smaller cut to 25 to 35 minutes total, basting twice. The pineapple rind can stay on.

NUTRITIONAL VALUE per serving	
Calories	562
Fat, total	26 g
Fat, saturated	10 g
Cholesterol	177 mg
Sodium	239 mg
Carbohydrate	12 g
Fiber	1 g
Protein	66 g
Calcium	29 mg
Iron	3 mg

Burritos

Makes 4 servings (2 per serving)

Tired of sandwiches? Here's a new idea for lunch or dinner! Extras can be warmed quickly in the microwave.

Tips

For instructions on cooking rice, see the cooking chart on page 46.

Make one large burrito (known as a Mexican pizza) by stacking tortillas alternately with filling ingedients.

2 tsp	vegetable oil	10 mL
2	cloves garlic, minced	2
1	small onion, chopped	1
1½ tsp	chili powder	7 mL
½ tsp	ground cumin	2 mL
1	can (19 oz/540 mL) pinto beans, rinsed and drained	1
1	can (12 oz/341 mL) corn kernels, drained	1
1½ cups	cooked brown rice	375 mL
½ cup	pitted black olives, sliced	125 mL
8	5½-inch (13.5 cm) GF corn tortillas	8
¾ cup	shredded lactose-free Cheddar cheese or Cheddar cheese	175 mL
2	green onions, thinly sliced	2
1	large tomato, diced	1
¼ cup	lactose-free plain yogurt or plain yogurt	50 mL
¾ cup	GF salsa	175 mL

1. In a large skillet, heat oil over medium-high heat. Add garlic, onion, chili powder and cumin; cook, stirring, for about 3 minutes, or until onion is tender. Stir in beans, corn, rice and olives. Reduce heat to medium and cook, stirring constantly, for 3 to 5 minutes, or until heated through.

2. Place one-eighth of the rice filling in the center of each tortilla. Top with cheese, green onions, tomato, yogurt and salsa. Fold the bottom third of the tortilla up over the filling. Fold the left side of the tortilla over the filling, then the right side. Roll up to enclose the filling in a neat, easy-to-eat packet.

Variation

Add grilled chicken breast strips or cooked ground beef. (For convenience, brown beef along with the onion and seasonings.)

NUTRITIONAL VALUE
per serving

Calories	558
Fat, total	15 g
Fat, saturated	2 g
Cholesterol	1 mg
Sodium	1,182 mg
Carbohydrate	85 g
Fiber	6 g
Protein	24 g
Calcium	277 mg
Iron	6 mg

Meatballs

How convenient to have meatballs at the ready when you're short on time! Just pop them frozen into a sauce to defrost and reheat at the same time.

Tips

We used Bread Sticks (page 224) to make the dry bread crumbs. For instructions on making bread crumbs, see the Technique Glossary, page 299.

Meatballs will be more tender if handled gently and not over-mixed.

Recipe can be doubled or tripled.

NUTRITIONAL VALUE per serving	
Calories	198
Fat, total	12 g
Fat, saturated	5 g
Cholesterol	74 mg
Sodium	195 mg
Carbohydrate	5 g
Fiber	0 g
Protein	16 g
Calcium	22 mg
Iron	2 mg

♦ *Preheat oven to 400°F (200°C)*
♦ *15- by 10-inch (40 by 25 cm) jelly-roll pan, lightly greased*

1 lb	lean ground beef	500 g
1	egg, slightly beaten	1
¼ cup	fine dry GF bread crumbs	50 mL
2 tbsp	snipped fresh oregano	25 mL
2 tbsp	tomato paste	25 mL
½ tsp	salt	2 mL
¼ tsp	freshly ground black pepper	1 mL

1. In a large bowl, combine ground beef, egg, bread crumbs, oregano, tomato paste, salt and pepper, mixing gently with a fork. Shape into 1-inch (2.5 cm) balls. Place in a single layer in prepared pan.

2. Bake in preheated oven for 15 to 20 minutes, or until no longer pink in the center. Let cool slightly, then freeze meatballs in the jellyroll pan. Once frozen, transfer meatballs to a heavy-duty freezer bag and seal bag. Freeze for up to 2 months.

3. *To serve:* Reheat meatballs from frozen directly in a sauce or place in a single layer on a plate and microwave on Low (30%) just until thawed, then add to a sauce.

To make this recipe egg-free

Omit egg from recipe. Combine 2 tbsp (25 mL) flax flour or ground flaxseed with 2 tbsp (25 mL) warm water. Let stand for 5 minutes. Add with tomato paste. Meatballs made this way tend to be slightly more tender, but they're fragile, so handle carefully.

Variation

Vary the seasoning to suit the sauce you plan to use. For example, use hot pepper flakes and cumin if you plan to use barbecue sauce; basil or sage for tomato sauce; or ground ginger for soy sauce.

Mini Meatloaves

**Makes
12 mini loaves
(2 per serving)**

Everybody has a meatloaf recipe, but why not try our moist, flavorful, egg-free version?

Tip

Mini meatloaves will be more tender if handled gently and not over-mixed.

◆ *Preheat oven to 400°F (200°C)*
◆ *12-cup muffin tin, lightly greased*
◆ *Rimmed baking sheet*

¾ cup	GF oats	175 mL
⅓ cup	fortified soy beverage, lactose-free milk or milk	75 mL
2 tbsp	ground flaxseed	25 mL
¼ cup	warm water	50 mL
2	onions, finely chopped	2
1 cup	diced mushrooms	250 mL
2 tbsp	grainy Dijon mustard	25 mL
2 tsp	dried thyme	10 mL
½ tsp	salt	2 mL
¼ tsp	freshly ground black pepper	1 mL
1 lb	lean ground beef	500 g
8 oz	lean ground pork	250 g

1. In a large bowl, combine oats and soy beverage; let stand for 10 minutes.

2. In a small bowl, combine flaxseed and warm water; let stand for 5 minutes. Add to oats. Add onions, mushrooms, mustard, thyme, salt and pepper; mix well. Using a fork, gently mix in beef and pork.

3. Spoon mixture evenly into each cup of prepared muffin tin, packing lightly. Place muffin tin on baking sheet, as it may bubble over.

4. Bake in preheated oven for 20 to 25 minutes, or until a meat thermometer inserted in a mini loaf registers 160°F (71°C) and meat is no longer pink inside. Let cooked mini meatloaves stand for 5 to 10 minutes. Remove from tin, draining off excess liquid.

NUTRITIONAL VALUE
per serving

Calories	362
Fat, total	22 g
Fat, saturated	8 g
Cholesterol	70 mg
Sodium	401 mg
Carbohydrate	16 g
Fiber	3 g
Protein	25 g
Calcium	64 mg
Iron	5 mg

Tips

For information on GF oats, see pages 37–39.

For more information on mushrooms, see page 117.

Variations

Make 1 large meatloaf. Spoon meat mixture into a 9- by 5-inch (2 L) loaf pan and bake at 400°F (200°C) for 60 to 75 minutes, or until a meat thermometer registers 160°F (71°C) and meat is no longer pink inside.

For individual shepherd's pies, use two 12-cup muffin tins. Spoon meat mixture evenly into 16 to 18 of the cups and top each with mashed potatoes before baking. Fill the empty cups three-quarters full with water.

Substitute marjoram for the thyme.

Fresh Mushrooms

Choose fresh, smooth mushrooms without large blemishes. The surface should be dry, but not dried out. They should have a firm texture, even color and tightly closed caps. Avoid discolored, broken and damaged mushrooms with soft spots.

A closed veil (the thin membrane under the cap) indicates a delicate flavor; an open veil means a richer flavor. Visible gills are an indication of age; the mushrooms are likely past their prime.

Refrigerate mushrooms in a paper bag and use within 3 days of purchase. Do not clean until ready to use. Always remove the plastic overlay from packaged mushrooms, and avoid airtight containers; moisture condensation speeds spoilage.

Clean mushrooms just before use. They are porous and absorb water like a sponge, so do not soak them. Instead, wipe them with a damp cloth or give them a quick rinse in cool water, then pat dry with paper towels.

Fresh mushrooms don't freeze well; however, sautéed mushrooms can be frozen for up to 1 month. After sautéing them, let them cool, then pack them into an airtight container.

Pasta Meatball Stew

This stew is colorful, nutritious and delicious. Better yet, it's easy to make, using meatballs straight from the freezer.

Tip

If the carrots are quite thick, cut them in half lengthwise so that all vegetables will cook in the same time.

1 tbsp	extra-virgin olive oil	15 mL
1	onion, chopped	1
3	cloves garlic, minced	3
2 tbsp	amaranth flour	25 mL
2 cups	GF beef stock	500 mL
1	can (28 oz /796 mL) whole tomatoes, drained	1
2 tbsp	tomato paste	25 mL
2 to 3 tbsp	snipped fresh oregano	25 to 45 mL
16	baby carrots	16
1	red bell pepper, cut into ¾-inch (2 cm) pieces	1
1½ cups	broccoli florets	375 mL
1	small zucchini, cut into 1-inch (2.5 cm) slices	1
1	batch Meatballs (see recipe, page 105)	1
1 cup	GF penne	250 mL
	Freshly ground black pepper	

1. In a large saucepan, heat olive oil over medium heat. Add onion and garlic; cook, stirring frequently, for 3 to 5 minutes, or until tender. Add amaranth flour; cook, stirring constantly, for 1 to 2 minutes. Gradually stir in stock, tomatoes, tomato paste and oregano to taste. Increase heat to medium-high and bring to a boil. Reduce heat to medium-low. Add carrots, bell pepper and broccoli; simmer for 15 minutes. Add zucchini and cooked meatballs and simmer for 10 minutes, or until vegetables are tender-crisp and meatballs are heated through.

2. Meanwhile, cook pasta according to package directions, or just until tender. Drain well and rinse under cold running water. Stir into stew and heat through. Season to taste with pepper.

NUTRITIONAL VALUE per serving	
Calories	352
Fat, total	15 g
Fat, saturated	5 g
Cholesterol	74 mg
Sodium	683 mg
Carbohydrate	25 g
Fiber	5 g
Protein	22 g
Calcium	122 mg
Iron	5 mg

Tip

When cooked, amaranth flour browns and looks like dried sand. Smell the aroma and enjoy the nutty flavor.

Variations

Substitute GF rotini or elbow macaroni for the penne.

Try different vegetables, such as fiddleheads, green beans, lima beans, okra, baby corn, celery and parsnips. Use a total of 3 cups (750 mL).

If time is short, steam the fresh vegetables or add a cooked vegetable mixture and simmer for 5 minutes with the meatballs.

Percentage of Fat in Ground Beef

U.S. standards

Until a final decision is made regarding the labeling of ground beef, consumers will have to continue to make their purchase decisions based on what is available in their supermarket. Generally, super-lean ground beef contains 7% to 10% fat; extra-lean ground beef (ground round) contains 15% fat; lean ground beef (ground chuck) contains 20% fat; and regular ground beef contains 30% fat. For more information, visit www.nal.usda.gov/fnic/foodcomp.

Canadian standards

Federal government regulations stipulate that ground beef labeled "extra-lean" may contain no more than 10% fat; "lean" may contain no more than 17% fat; "medium" may contain no more than 23% fat; and "regular" may contain no more than 30% fat. For more information, visit www.beefinfo.org.

Tomato Pasta Sauce

**Makes 6 cups
(1.5 L)
(1 cup/250 mL
per serving)**

Fresh tomato season
never lasts long enough.
Purchase tomatoes in
bulk and double or
triple this recipe to
freeze, ready for a
variety of quick and easy
mid-week dinners.

Tips

Purchase 1½ lbs (750 g)
Roma (plum) or beefsteak
tomatoes. There are
9 Roma tomatoes or
3 medium beefsteak
tomatoes in 1 lb (500 g).

For information on
removing seeds from
tomatoes, see the
Technique Glossary,
page 302.

1 tsp	extra-virgin olive oil	5 mL
3	cloves garlic, minced	3
1	onion, chopped	1
⅓ cup	fresh rosemary, snipped	75 mL
½ cup	dry red wine	125 mL
3 cups	chopped seeded peeled tomatoes	750 mL
¼ cup	capers, well drained	50 mL
2	bay leaves	2
1 tsp	grated lemon zest	5 mL

1. In a large saucepan, heat olive oil over medium heat.
Add garlic, onion and rosemary; cook, stirring, for
5 minutes, or until tender. Slowly add wine, then
add tomatoes, capers, bay leaves and lemon zest;
bring to a boil. Reduce heat to medium-low and
simmer, stirring occasionally, for about 1 hour, or
until thickened. Remove bay leaves before serving.

Variations

Substitute 2 cans (each 28 oz/796 mL) whole
tomatoes, with juice, for the fresh.

Substitute GF vegetable stock for the wine.

NUTRITIONAL VALUE per serving	
Calories	64
Fat, total	1 g
Fat, saturated	0 g
Cholesterol	0 mg
Sodium	214 mg
Carbohydrate	8 g
Fiber	2 g
Protein	2 g
Calcium	56 mg
Iron	2 mg

Side Dishes

Grilled Vegetable Platter

Makes 4 servings

This all-purpose recipe can easily be doubled, tripled or halved to suit the size of the group.

Tip

If you have a roasting basket for the outdoor grill, bell peppers can be cut smaller.

◆ Barbecue, preheated to high

⅓ cup	extra-virgin olive oil	75 mL
3 tbsp	balsamic vinegar	45 mL
4	cloves garlic, minced	4
12	asparagus spears, trimmed	12
2	portobello mushrooms, stems removed	2
2	green onions, trimmed	2
1	small Italian eggplant, cut crosswise into ½-inch (1 cm) slices	1
1	red bell pepper, cut into eighths	1
1	yellow bell pepper, cut into eighths	1
½	large red onion, cut into ½-inch (1 cm) slices	½

1. In a large bowl, whisk together olive oil, vinegar and garlic. Add asparagus, mushrooms, green onions, eggplant, red and yellow peppers and red onion. Stir to coat well.

2. Reduce barbecue heat to medium. Grill vegetables, beginning with eggplant and peppers and adding remaining vegetables according to their required cooking times (see below), turning occasionally, until tender.

   - Eggplant, red and yellow peppers: 20 minutes
   - Red onion, mushrooms: 15 minutes
   - Asparagus, green onions: 8 minutes

NUTRITIONAL VALUE
per serving

Calories	332
Fat, total	25 g
Fat, saturated	3 g
Cholesterol	0 mg
Sodium	158 mg
Carbohydrate	23 g
Fiber	6 g
Protein	5 g
Calcium	44 mg
Iron	1 mg

Variations

Substitute 4 oyster mushrooms for the portobellos.

Refrigerate grilled vegetables overnight to serve as a salad the next day.

To use an indoor (contact) grill, grill eggplant. Remove and set aside to keep warm while grilling the remaining vegetables. Vegetables cook faster than on a barbecue.

Ratatouille

Makes 4 servings

This vegetable ragoût from the French region of Provence is made with tomatoes, eggplant, zucchini and bell pepper. Our version features our Tomato Pasta Sauce (page 110).

Tips

Choose a firm, smooth-skinned eggplant that feels heavy for its size. It should give a little when pressed.

If the sauce is too thick, add a small amount of dry red wine or GF vegetable stock.

2 tsp	extra-virgin olive oil	10 mL
2	cloves garlic, minced	2
1	Italian eggplant, cut into ½-inch (1 cm) slices	1
1	yellow bell pepper, cut into ¼-inch (0.5 cm) strips	1
1	small zucchini, cut into ½-inch (1 cm) slices	1
1½ cups	Tomato Pasta Sauce (see recipe, page 110)	375 mL

1. In a large skillet, heat olive oil over medium heat. Add garlic, eggplant, yellow pepper and zucchini; cook, stirring frequently, for 8 to 10 minutes, or until tender. Add pasta sauce and simmer until hot.

Variations

If an Italian eggplant is not available, use a regular eggplant and cut the slices into quarters.

Add or substitute cooked green beans, fennel, mushrooms or carrots.

If you don't have a batch of Tomato Pasta Sauce ready to go, you can use a commercial GF tomato pasta sauce.

NUTRITIONAL VALUE per serving	
Calories	93
Fat, total	3 g
Fat, saturated	0 g
Cholesterol	0 mg
Sodium	168 mg
Carbohydrate	14 g
Fiber	1 g
Protein	3 g
Calcium	42 mg
Iron	1 mg

Roasted Asparagus with Hazelnuts

Makes 4 to 6 servings

This versatile spring vegetable, now available year-round, makes an excellent side dish served hot or chilled.

Tip

Don't overcook asparagus. Roast just until fork-tender.

♦ *Preheat oven to 450°F (220°C)*
♦ *15- by 10-inch (40 by 25 cm) jelly-roll pan, ungreased*

2	cloves garlic, minced	2
½ cup	extra-virgin olive oil	125 mL
1½ lbs	fresh asparagus spears, trimmed	750 g
½ cup	sliced hazelnuts	125 mL
¼ cup	red wine vinegar	50 mL
	Salt and freshly ground black pepper	

1. In the jelly-roll pan, whisk together garlic and olive oil. Add asparagus. Using your fingers, roll asparagus to coat evenly. Arrange asparagus in pan in a single layer. Sprinkle with hazelnuts.

2. Roast in preheated oven for 10 to 12 minutes, or until tender-crisp. Drizzle with vinegar and toss gently to coat. Season with salt and pepper to taste. Serve immediately.

Variation

For a cold salad, refrigerate roasted asparagus overnight before serving.

Asparagus

Select firm, plump spears with tightly closed tips. The full length of the spear should be a bright green color. Store asparagus upright in the refrigerator in ½ inch (1 cm) of water or with the ends wrapped in a moist paper towel. It should not be washed until just before use. Don't cut asparagus spears while cleaning — simply bend the spear and snap off the woody end at the natural breaking point.

NUTRITIONAL VALUE per serving	
Calories	256
Fat, total	24 g
Fat, saturated	3 g
Cholesterol	0 mg
Sodium	3 mg
Carbohydrate	7 g
Fiber	3 g
Protein	4 g
Calcium	41 mg
Iron	2 mg

Caramelized Peppers and Onions with Pasta

Makes 4 servings

Enjoy this colorful, tasty, modern spin on traditional Italian peppers and onions. Just add cooked meat or seafood to complete the meal.

Tips

Don't rush this dish — the more the vegetables caramelize, the deeper the flavor.

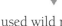

We used wild rice fusilli for the pasta, but you can use any kind you like.

♦ 9- to 10-inch (23 to 25 cm) skillet, 2 inches (5 cm) deep

2 tsp	extra-virgin olive oil	10 mL
3	red bell peppers, cut into ¼-inch (0.5 cm) slices	3
3	cloves garlic, minced	3
2	Vidalia or other sweet onions, thinly sliced	2
1 tsp	liquid honey	5 mL
¼ cup	snipped fresh parsley	50 mL
2 tbsp	snipped fresh oregano	25 mL
¼ cup	balsamic vinegar	50 mL
	Salt and freshly ground black pepper	
2 cups	GF pasta	500 mL

1. In a large nonstick skillet, heat olive oil over low heat. Add peppers, garlic, onions and honey; cover and cook, stirring occasionally, for 15 to 20 minutes, or until tender and deep golden brown. Remove from heat and stir in parsley, oregano and vinegar. Season to taste with salt and pepper.

2. Meanwhile, cook pasta according to package directions, or just until tender. Drain well. Toss with caramelized peppers and onions.

Variation

To turn this recipe into a complete entrée, add a protein (such as two 6-oz/170 g cans of tuna, drained, or 12 oz/375 g cooked sliced GF Italian sausage) when tossing vegetables with pasta.

NUTRITIONAL VALUE per serving	
Calories	237
Fat, total	4 g
Fat, saturated	1 g
Cholesterol	0 mg
Sodium	29 mg
Carbohydrate	47 g
Fiber	3 g
Protein	5 g
Calcium	67 mg
Iron	2 mg

Mushroom and Sweet Potato Casserole

Makes 4 servings

The next time you're thinking of making scalloped potatoes, try this more nutritious version instead.

Tip

To make ahead: Bake, covered, without topping, for 50 to 55 minutes, or until potatoes are fork-tender. Let cool, cover and refrigerate for up to 3 days. Reheat in the microwave, then sprinkle with topping and place under preheated broiler until topping is browned and crisp.

♦ *Preheat oven to 350°F (180°C)*
♦ *6-cup (1.5 L) baking dish with lid, lightly greased*

1 tsp	vegetable oil	5 mL
1	onion, chopped	1
2 cups	sliced mixed mushrooms (shiitake, button and/or cremini)	500 mL
¼ cup	snipped fresh rosemary	50 mL
1	large sweet potato, peeled and very thinly sliced	1
½	small butternut squash, peeled and very thinly sliced	½
⅔ cup	GF vegetable stock	150 mL

Topping

½ cup	GF fresh bread crumbs	125 mL
¼ cup	grated lactose-free Parmesan cheese or Parmesan cheese	50 mL
2 tbsp	snipped fresh rosemary	25 mL
2 tbsp	lactose-free buttery spread or butter, melted	25 mL

1. In a skillet, heat oil over medium heat. Add onion and cook, stirring, for 2 to 3 minutes, or until tender. Increase heat to medium-high and add mushrooms. Cook, stirring frequently, for 3 to 5 minutes, or until well browned. Stir in rosemary. Remove from heat.

2. In prepared baking dish, layer potato and squash slices alternately with mushroom mixture, making 3 layers of potato and squash and 2 layers of mushroom mixture. Pour stock over vegetables.

3. Cover tightly and bake in preheated oven for 30 minutes.

NUTRITIONAL VALUE
per serving

Calories	222
Fat, total	9 g
Fat, saturated	5 g
Cholesterol	8 mg
Sodium	340 mg
Carbohydrate	31 g
Fiber	4 g
Protein	6 g
Calcium	61 mg
Iron	3 mg

Tip

For more information on mushrooms, see page 107.

4. *Meanwhile, prepare the topping:* In a small bowl, combine bread crumbs, Parmesan cheese, rosemary and buttery spread.

5. Remove lid and sprinkle topping evenly over vegetables. Bake, uncovered, for 20 to 25 minutes, or until vegetables are fork-tender.

Variations

Substitute another winter squash, such as Hubbard, acorn, pepper or turban.

Substitute 2 carrots, sliced into thin coins, for the squash.

More About Mushrooms

- Button (white, agaricus) mushrooms are the most common mushrooms and are available fresh, canned or dried. They range from creamy white to beige. The smooth, round, small ones have closed veils (the gills on the underside are covered), while the larger ones have open veils. Their mild, woodsy flavor intensifies upon cooking.
- Cremini (brown, Italian) mushrooms are related to button mushrooms, but have light tan to brown caps. They have a more intense, earthier flavor and a very firm texture. Cremini mushrooms can be substituted for button mushrooms.
- Shiitake (oak, Chinese black, forest) mushrooms have broad, umbrella-shaped caps up to 10 inches (25 cm) in diameter, with wide-open veils and tan gills. They range from tan to dark brown. Shiitakes are soft and spongy in texture, with a full, woodsy flavor. They should be cooked thoroughly for a meaty texture. The woody stems are removed and used in soup stock.

Wild Rice Latkes

Makes 12 to 14 latkes (1 per serving)

We've added wild and brown rice to a traditional Jewish pancake. No need to wait for Hanukkah to serve these crisp golden rice and potato cakes. Serve as appetizers or as a side to a main course.

Tips

Select a high-starch potato variety, such as Yukon gold or russet.

To grate potatoes, use the grating disk of a food processor or the coarse side of a box grater.

Remove any small cooked bits from the skillet between batches, if necessary.

NUTRITIONAL VALUE per serving

Calories	42
Fat, total	1 g
Fat, saturated	0 g
Cholesterol	13 mg
Sodium	89 mg
Carbohydrate	8 g
Fiber	1 g
Protein	2 g
Calcium	18 mg
Iron	1 mg

◆ *Preheat oven to 250°F (120°C)*
◆ *Baking sheet, lined with paper towels*

2 cups	grated potatoes (unpeeled)	500 mL
1	onion, finely chopped	1
½ cup	long-grain or short-grain brown rice, cooked and cooled	125 mL
½ cup	wild rice, cooked and cooled	125 mL
1	egg, beaten	1
3 tbsp	amaranth flour	45 mL
½ tsp	GF baking powder	2 mL
½ tsp	salt	2 mL
	Vegetable oil for frying	

1. In a sieve set over the sink or a bowl, combine potatoes and onion. Using your hands, firmly squeeze handfuls of grated potatoes to get rid of as much liquid as possible. Transfer to a large bowl and add brown rice, wild rice, egg, amaranth flour, baking powder and salt. Mix well.

2. In a large skillet, over medium-high heat, heat just enough oil to cover the bottom of the pan in a thin layer. In batches, using 2 tbsp (25 mL) of the mixture per latke, drop latkes about 1 inch (2.5 cm) apart in pan. Flatten to ¼ inch (0.5 cm) thickness with the back of a spoon. Fry for 3 to 5 minutes per side, using 2 spatulas to turn latkes once, until crisp and golden. Drain on prepared baking sheet. Place in preheated oven to keep warm.

3. Repeat with remaining mixture, adding oil and reheating pan between batches as needed. Serve hot.

> **To make this recipe egg-free**
> Omit egg from recipe. Combine 2 tbsp (25 mL) flax flour or ground flaxseed with ¼ cup (50 mL) warm water. Mix together. Let stand for 5 minutes. Mix in with vegetables and rice.

Tip

To make ahead: Fry latkes and place on prepared baking sheet to cool. Stack between layers of waxed paper in an airtight container. Refrigerate for up to 3 days or freeze up to 1 month. To reheat, defrost overnight in the refrigerator (if frozen). Bake cold latkes in a single layer, uncovered, in center of a 400°F (200°C) oven for 5 minutes. Using 2 spatulas, turn latkes over. Continue baking for 5 to 8 minutes, or until crisp. Serve immediately.

Variations

Substitute short-grain white rice for the brown rice.

Pass an assortment of toppings, such as lactose-free sour cream, lactose-free yogurt, applesauce, smoked salmon, capers and chives.

Great Latkes

- To ensure crisp latkes, be sure to squeeze excess water from potatoes before mixing. The drier they are, the less likely they are to break during frying.
- For a fluffy latke, don't grate the onion, just thinly slice.
- Use only small amounts of latke batter; larger amounts tend to absorb more oil during frying.
- Test the temperature of the oil by adding a small amount of latke batter; it should turn golden in 1 to 2 minutes.

Coconut Rice

Makes 4 servings

This sticky rice is the perfect accompaniment to Coconut Shrimp (page 92) or as the base for a stir-fry!

Tips

Be sure to shake the can of coconut milk well to mix before using.

If using regular (higher fat) coconut milk, use ³⁄₄ cup (175 mL) coconut milk and ¹⁄₂ cup (125 mL) water.

¹⁄₂ cup	jasmine rice	125 mL
1¹⁄₄ cups	light coconut milk	300 mL
¹⁄₄ cup	chopped red onion	50 mL
1	clove garlic, minced	1
1 tsp	ground ginger	5 mL
¹⁄₄ cup	raisins	50 mL
¹⁄₄ cup	peanuts	50 mL
	Salt	

1. In a sieve, rinse rice under cold running water until water runs fairly clear. Drain.

2. In a medium saucepan, combine rice, coconut milk, onion, garlic and ginger. Bring to a boil over medium heat. Reduce heat to low, cover and simmer gently for 20 minutes, or until rice is tender and most of the liquid is absorbed. Remove from heat and let stand for 5 minutes. Stir in raisins, peanuts and salt to taste. Fluff with a fork.

Variations

Substitute basmati, Arborio or short-grain white rice for the jasmine rice. See "Cooking Rice," page 46, for cooking times.

Use ¹⁄₂ cup (125 mL) of either raisins or peanuts.

NUTRITIONAL VALUE per serving	
Calories	251
Fat, total	12 g
Fat, saturated	8 g
Cholesterol	0 mg
Sodium	21 mg
Carbohydrate	32 g
Fiber	2 g
Protein	6 g
Calcium	39 mg
Iron	2 mg

Wild Rice with Blueberries

Makes 6 servings

Serve this colorful and attractive side with roast duck, Cornish game hen or venison.

Tips

This side can be made up to 2 days ahead, chilled and reheated.

We like to make this quantity and freeze in meal-size portions (it can be frozen for up to 4 weeks), but the recipe can be halved.

For information on mushrooms, see pages 107 and 117.

½ cup	wild rice	125 mL
3 cups	GF vegetable stock	750 mL
1 cup	chopped onions	250 mL
2 cups	sliced mushrooms	500 mL
½ cup	dried blueberries	125 mL
½ cup	chopped hazelnuts	125 mL
1 tbsp	snipped fresh rosemary	15 mL
Pinch	freshly ground black pepper	Pinch

1. In a sieve, rinse wild rice under cold running water; drain well. In a large saucepan, combine rice, vegetable stock and onions. Bring to a boil over high heat. Reduce heat to medium-low and simmer, uncovered, for 35 minutes. Stir in mushrooms, blueberries, hazelnuts, rosemary and pepper. Cover and simmer for 10 minutes, or until rice is soft but not mushy and liquid is absorbed. Serve hot.

Variations

Substitute GF beef or chicken stock for the GF vegetable stock. Either use a homemade stock or reconstitute a commercial GF stock powder.

Substitute brown rice for half the wild rice.

For richer flavor, use a variety of mushrooms, which could include cremini, portobello, portobellini or shiitake.

NUTRITIONAL VALUE per serving	
Calories	124
Fat, total	1 g
Fat, saturated	0 g
Cholesterol	0 mg
Sodium	363 mg
Carbohydrate	25 g
Fiber	4 g
Protein	4 g
Calcium	31 mg
Iron	1 mg

Asparagus Risotto

Makes 4 to 6 servings

Our version of risotto is packed with fresh vegetables, and the method is streamlined for today's busy lifestyle. Serve as an accompaniment to lamb, salmon or ham.

Tips

Serve immediately to keep the creamy texture.

For more information on asparagus, see page 114.

1 lb	asparagus	500 g
2 tsp	extra-virgin olive oil	10 mL
2	cloves garlic, minced	2
1	onion, chopped	1
1	yellow bell pepper, cut into 1-inch (2.5 cm) pieces	1
1 cup	baby carrots, sliced in half lengthwise	250 mL
1 cup	Arborio rice	250 mL
1½ cups	GF vegetable stock	375 mL
½ cup	dry white wine	125 mL
1 tsp	dried rosemary	5 mL
	Salt and freshly ground white pepper	

1. Bend asparagus spears and snap off woody ends at the natural breaking point. Cut spears into 1-inch (2.5 cm) pieces; set stalks and tips aside separately.

2. In a large pot, heat olive oil over medium heat. Add garlic, onion, bell pepper, carrots and rice. Cook, stirring, for 5 to 7 minutes, or until vegetables are soft. Stir in stock, wine, rosemary and asparagus stalks (reserving tender tips). Bring to a boil. Reduce heat to medium-low, cover and simmer for 10 minutes. Quickly add tender asparagus tips on top, without stirring. Cover and simmer for 10 minutes, or until rice is tender and liquid is absorbed. Season to taste with salt and pepper.

NUTRITIONAL VALUE per serving	
Calories	179
Fat, total	2 g
Fat, saturated	0 g
Cholesterol	0 mg
Sodium	193 mg
Carbohydrate	35 g
Fiber	2 g
Protein	5 g
Calcium	44 mg
Iron	1 mg

Variations

Substitute any short-grain rice for the Arborio rice.

Substitute quinoa for all or part of the rice.

If you prefer not to use white wine, increase the GF stock to 2 cups (500 mL).

For a creamier, more traditional risotto, increase the amount of liquid to up to 5 cups (1.25 L). Cook, uncovered, adding 1 cup (250 mL) stock at a time, stirring frequently and allowing all stock to be absorbed before adding more.

Cilantro Romano Pilaf

Makes 5 servings

Serve as a vegetarian main dish or as a side with chicken or fish. It's also great as the filling in a burrito made from a GF corn tortilla.

Tips

Leave the peel on the zucchini for an attractive color combo.

Choose a long-grain rice that stays as individual grains rather than clumping together.

1 tsp	vegetable oil	5 mL
½	small onion, chopped	½
1	clove garlic, minced	1
½ cup	long-grain brown rice	125 mL
¼ cup	drained oil-packed sun-dried tomatoes, chopped	50 mL
2 tbsp	fresh cilantro, snipped	25 mL
1½ cups	GF vegetable stock	375 mL
1 cup	drained rinsed canned Romano beans (about half a 19-oz/540 mL can)	250 mL
½	small zucchini, cut into ½-inch (1 cm) slices	½
	Salt and freshly ground black pepper	

1. In a large saucepan, heat oil over medium heat. Cook onion and garlic, stirring, for about 3 minutes, or until tender. Add rice, sun-dried tomatoes, cilantro and stock; bring to a boil. Reduce heat to low, cover and simmer gently for 45 minutes. Sprinkle beans and zucchini over rice, without stirring. Cover and cook for 5 to 7 minutes, or until rice is tender, liquid is absorbed and beans are hot. Season to taste with salt and pepper. Fluff with a fork.

Variation

Substitute quinoa or white rice for the brown rice and adjust the simmering time according to package directions.

NUTRITIONAL VALUE per serving	
Calories	140
Fat, total	3 g
Fat, saturated	0 g
Cholesterol	0 mg
Sodium	343 mg
Carbohydrate	25 g
Fiber	4 g
Protein	5 g
Calcium	32 mg
Iron	1 mg

Cranberry Walnut Quinoa Pilaf

Makes 6 servings

Serve this tasty side dish with Rubbed Roast Chicken (page 96). Just add a salad to complete your supper menu.

Tips

See the Technique Glossary, page 301, for instructions on toasting nuts.

Quinoa is cooked when grains turn from white to transparent and the tiny, spiral-like germ is separated.

2 tsp	extra-virgin olive oil	10 mL
½ cup	chopped onion	125 mL
1	stalk celery, diced	1
½ cup	quinoa, rinsed	125 mL
1½ cups	GF vegetable stock	375 mL
½ cup	dried cranberries	125 mL
1 tbsp	dried tarragon	15 mL
	Salt and freshly ground black pepper	
⅓ cup	coarsely chopped toasted walnuts	75 mL
1	red-skinned, firm-textured apple, diced	1
2	green onions, green tops only, chopped	2

1. In a large saucepan, heat olive oil over medium-low heat. Add onion and celery and cook, stirring frequently, for 6 to 8 minutes, or until tender. Add quinoa, stock, cranberries and tarragon; increase heat and bring to a boil. Reduce heat to low, cover and simmer gently for 18 to 20 minutes, or until quinoa is tender and liquid is absorbed. Season to taste with salt and pepper. Stir in walnuts, apple and green onions.

Variations

Substitute diced dried apricots, dried blueberries or currants for the dried cranberries.

Substitute long-grain brown rice for the quinoa. Refer to package directions or "Cooking Rice," page 46, for the quantity of GF stock to use and cooking times.

NUTRITIONAL VALUE per serving	
Calories	169
Fat, total	7 g
Fat, saturated	1 g
Cholesterol	0 mg
Sodium	193 mg
Carbohydrate	24 g
Fiber	3 g
Protein	4 g
Calcium	41 mg
Iron	2 mg

Autumn Quinoa Casserole

Makes 6 servings

High-protein quinoa makes an interesting alternative to rice and other grains. In this dish, the grains are toasted to give a pleasant, nutty taste. Serve as an accompaniment to grilled meats or poultry, or on its own.

Tips

Don't skip the toasting and browning of the rice and quinoa, as this enriches the flavor.

Dice the carrot slightly smaller than the squash so it will take the same amount of time to cook.

* *Preheat oven to 375°F (190°C)*
* *8- to 10-cup (2 to 2.5 L) baking dish with lid, ungreased*

¼ cup	long-grain brown rice	50 mL
¼ cup	quinoa	50 mL
½	small onion, diced	½
1	clove garlic, minced	1
1 cup	diced peeled butternut squash	250 mL
1 cup	diced carrot	250 mL
1 tbsp	grated orange zest	15 mL
½ cup	orange juice	125 mL
1½ cups	GF vegetable stock	375 mL
1 tsp	dried sage	5 mL
1 tsp	dried savory	5 mL
¼ cup	chopped fresh parsley	50 mL
	Salt and freshly ground black pepper	

1. In a large skillet, over medium-high heat, cook brown rice and quinoa, stirring constantly, for 8 to 10 minutes, or until lightly toasted and browned. Remove from heat.

2. In baking dish, combine onion, garlic, squash, carrot, orange juice and stock. Stir in rice, quinoa, sage and savory.

3. Cover and bake in preheated oven for 50 minutes. Uncover and bake for about 10 minutes, or until grains and vegetables are tender and liquid is absorbed. Fluff with a fork. Stir in parsley and orange zest. Season to taste with salt and pepper.

Variations

Substitute apple juice for the orange juice.

Substitute extra quinoa for the brown rice.

NUTRITIONAL VALUE per serving	
Calories	93
Fat, total	1 g
Fat, saturated	0 g
Cholesterol	0 mg
Sodium	194 mg
Carbohydrate	20 g
Fiber	2 g
Protein	3 g
Calcium	42 mg
Iron	1 mg

Mock Soy Sauce

If you are having trouble finding GF soy sauce in your area, try our soy-free version.

1½ cups	boiling water	375 mL
3	GF beef bouillon cubes (or 3 tbsp/45 mL GF beef stock powder)	3
¼ cup	cider vinegar	50 mL
2 tbsp	sesame oil	25 mL
2 tbsp	fancy molasses	25 mL
Pinch	freshly ground black pepper	Pinch

1. Dissolve bouillon cubes in boiling water. Gradually whisk in vinegar, sesame oil, molasses and pepper until blended. Store in a covered jar in the refrigerator for up to 1 month.

**NUTRITIONAL VALUE
per serving**

Calories	14
Fat, total	1 g
Fat, saturated	0 g
Cholesterol	0 mg
Sodium	119 mg
Carbohydrate	1 g
Fiber	0 g
Protein	0 g
Calcium	7 mg
Iron	0 mg

Yeast-Free Biscuits, Muffins and Loaves

Extra Baking Tips for Biscuits, Muffins and Loaves

- The batters should be the same consistency as wheat flour batters, but you can mix them more without producing tough products, full of tunnels.
- Use a portion scoop to quickly divide the batter into muffin cups to ensure muffins are equal in size and bake in the same length of time.
- When baking one of the recipes that yields 6 muffins, if you don't have a 6-cup muffin tin, use a 12-cup tin and half-fill the empty cups with water before baking.
- Bake in muffin tins of a different size. Mini muffins take 12 to 15 minutes to bake, while jumbo muffins bake in 20 to 40 minutes. Check jumbo muffins for doneness after 20 minutes, then again every 5 to 10 minutes. Keep in mind that the baking time will vary with the amount of batter in each muffin cup.
- Fill muffin tins and loaf pans no more than three-quarters full. Let batter-filled pans stand for 30 minutes for a more tender product. It's worth the wait. We set a timer for 20 minutes, then preheat the oven so both the oven and the batter are ready at the same time.
- If muffins stick to the lightly greased tins, let stand for a minute or two and try again. Loosen with a spatula, if necessary.
- Muffins and biscuits can be reheated in the microwave, wrapped in a paper towel, for a few seconds on Medium (50%) power.
- To freeze, place individual muffins or loaf slices in small freezer bags, then place all in a large airtight freezer plastic bag. Freeze for up to 1 month.

Working with Biscuit Mix

- Stir the mix before spooning very lightly into the dry measures when dividing into portions in Step 2 of method. Do not pack.
- Be sure to divide the mix into 8 equal portions before using to make up an individual recipe. Depending on how much air you incorporate into the mix and the texture of the individual gluten-free flours, the total volume of the mix can vary slightly. The important thing is to make 8 equal portions.
- Label and date packages before storing. We add the page number of the recipe to the label as a quick reference.
- Let warm to room temperature and mix well before using.
- Mix can be halved to make 4 batches of 6 biscuits each.
- If you prefer to make a dozen biscuits at a time, divide the mix into 4 equal portions of approximately $2\frac{1}{2}$ cups (625 mL) and double all the ingredients listed in the individual biscuit recipes.

Biscuit Mix

Makes 10 cups (2.5 L), or enough for 8 batches of 6 biscuits each (1 biscuit per serving)

Crave hot, homemade, melt-in-your-mouth biscuits? Choose any one of the four variations found on the following pages. Have this mix ready to quickly whip up a batch for breakfast, lunch or dinner. They'll disappear right before your eyes.

Tip

Select a shortening that is low in trans fat, if available in your area.

2 cups	brown rice flour	500 mL
2 cups	sorghum flour	500 mL
1 cup	amaranth flour	250 mL
1 cup	tapioca starch	250 mL
½ cup	granulated sugar	125 mL
1 tbsp	xanthan gum	15 mL
¼ cup	GF baking powder	50 mL
1 tbsp	baking soda	15 mL
2 tsp	salt	10 mL
2 cups	shortening	500 mL

1. In a large bowl, combine brown rice flour, sorghum flour, amaranth flour, tapioca starch, sugar, xanthan gum, baking powder, baking soda and salt. Using a pastry blender or 2 knives, cut in shortening until mixture resembles coarse crumbs about the size of small peas.

2. Immediately divide into 8 equal portions of approximately 1¼ cups (300 mL) each. Seal tightly in plastic bags, removing as much air as possible. Store at room temperature for up to 3 days or freeze for up to 6 months.

NUTRITIONAL VALUE per serving	
Calories	148
Fat, total	9 g
Fat, saturated	2 g
Cholesterol	0 mg
Sodium	178 mg
Carbohydrate	16 g
Fiber	1 g
Protein	2 g
Calcium	61 mg
Iron	1 mg

Plain Jane Biscuits

Makes 6 biscuits (1 per serving)

For those who love their flavors pure and uncomplicated — a true plain Jane!

Tips

To reheat leftover biscuits, wrap loosely in a paper towel and microwave each biscuit at Medium (50%) power for a few seconds.

This is a great drop biscuit to top a stew or chili.

◆ *Preheat oven to 400°F (200°C)*
◆ *Baking sheet, lightly greased*

¼ cup	fortified soy beverage, lactose-free milk or milk	50 mL
1 tsp	freshly squeezed lemon juice	5 mL
1¼ cups	Biscuit Mix (see recipe, page 129)	300 mL

1. In a measuring cup or bowl, combine soy beverage and lemon juice; set aside for 5 minutes.
2. In a medium bowl, combine biscuit mix and soy beverage mixture, stirring with a fork or rubber spatula to make a soft, slightly sticky dough.
3. Drop by heaping spoonfuls onto prepared baking sheet.
4. Bake in preheated oven for 13 to 15 minutes, or until tops are golden. Serve immediately.

Variation

To turn these into shortcakes, add 1 tbsp (15 mL) granulated sugar to the biscuit mix. Top with fresh fruit in season.

NUTRITIONAL VALUE per serving	
Calories	153
Fat, total	9 g
Fat, saturated	2 g
Cholesterol	0 mg
Sodium	183 mg
Carbohydrate	16 g
Fiber	1 g
Protein	2 g
Calcium	73 mg
Iron	1 mg

Apricot Pecan Biscuits

Makes 8 biscuits (1 per serving)

With their flecks of golden apricots, these biscuits are a treat for the eye — and your taste buds! Serve them for dessert!

Tips

Look for applesauce in 4-oz (113 g) single-serving containers. We like the convenience of not having to open and quickly use up the larger jars.

You can use any of the many different flavors of applesauce. We liked the Apple Mango Peach fruit blend.

- ◆ *Preheat oven to 375°F (190°C)*
- ◆ *Baking sheet, lightly greased*

1¼ cups	Biscuit Mix (see recipe, page 129)	300 mL
¼ cup	pecan flour	50 mL
½ cup	snipped dried apricots	125 mL
¼ cup	chopped pecans, toasted	50 mL
1	4-oz (113 g) container unsweetened applesauce	1

1. In a medium bowl, combine biscuit mix, pecan flour, apricots and pecans. Add applesauce all at once, stirring with a fork or rubber spatula to make a soft, slightly sticky dough.

2. Drop by heaping spoonfuls onto prepared baking sheet.

3. Bake in preheated oven for 13 to 15 minutes, or until tops are golden. Serve immediately.

Variations

Replace half the apricots with the same quantity of dates.

Substitute either almond or hazelnut flour for the pecan flour and the appropriate nut for the pecans.

Pecan Storage

Protect from moisture, light, heat and air to keep fresh. Store in an airtight container to prevent absorption of moisture, gases and odors. In-shell pecans can be stored in a cool, dry place for 6 to 12 months. Shelled pecans can be kept in an airtight container in the refrigerator for up to 9 months or in a sealed plastic bag in the freezer for up to 2 years. Pecans can be thawed and refrozen without loss of flavor or texture.

NUTRITIONAL VALUE per serving	
Calories	186
Fat, total	12 g
Fat, saturated	2 g
Cholesterol	0 mg
Sodium	135 mg
Carbohydrate	20 g
Fiber	2 g
Protein	2 g
Calcium	54 mg
Iron	2 mg

Bacon and Tomato Biscuits

Makes 6 biscuits (1 per serving)

Enjoy the salty tang of this quick and easy savory biscuit hot from the oven.

Tip

Use dry, not oil-packed, sun-dried tomatoes. Snip soft sun-dried tomatoes into ¼-inch (0.5 cm) pieces for a stronger burst of tomato goodness.

♦ *Preheat oven to 400°F (200°C)*
♦ *Baking sheet, lightly greased*

¼ cup	fortified soy beverage, lactose-free milk or milk	50 mL
1 tsp	freshly squeezed lemon juice	5 mL
1¼ cups	Biscuit Mix (see recipe, page 129)	300 mL
3	slices GF bacon, cooked crisp and crumbled	3
¼ cup	snipped dry-packed sun-dried tomatoes	50 mL
1 tsp	dried basil	5 mL

1. In a measuring cup or bowl, combine soy beverage and lemon juice; set aside for 5 minutes.

2. In a medium bowl, combine biscuit mix, bacon, tomatoes and basil. Add soy beverage mixture all at once, stirring with a fork or rubber spatula to make a soft, slightly sticky dough.

3. Drop by heaping spoonfuls onto prepared baking sheet.

4. Bake in preheated oven for 13 to 15 minutes, or until tops are golden. Serve immediately.

Variations

Substitute sliced Kalamata olives for the bacon, and oregano or rosemary for the basil.

Substitute 1 tbsp (15 mL) snipped fresh basil for the dried.

NUTRITIONAL VALUE per serving

Calories	177
Fat, total	11 g
Fat, saturated	2 g
Cholesterol	3 mg
Sodium	281 mg
Carbohydrate	18 g
Fiber	1 g
Protein	3 g
Calcium	80 mg
Iron	2 mg

Orange Poppy Seed Biscuits

Makes 6 biscuits (1 per serving)

There's no rule that says lemon is the only flavor that combines well with poppy seeds — the proof is in these biscuits, which use fresh oranges.

Tips

Zest the whole orange and freeze any leftovers for the next time. Be careful not to include any of the bitter white part of the orange.

Real poppy seed lovers can double the amount stated in the recipe.

♦ Preheat oven to 375°F (190°C)
♦ Baking sheet, lightly greased

1¼ cups	Biscuit Mix (see recipe, page 129)	300 mL
1 tbsp	poppy seeds	15 mL
1 tbsp	grated orange zest	15 mL
¼ cup	freshly squeezed orange juice	50 mL

1. In a medium bowl, combine biscuit mix, poppy seeds and orange zest. Add orange juice all at once, stirring with a fork or rubber spatula to make a soft, slightly sticky dough.
2. Drop by heaping spoonfuls onto prepared baking sheet.
3. Bake in preheated oven for 13 to 15 minutes, or until tops are golden. Serve immediately.

Variation
Substitute lemon for the orange and add fresh rosemary and freshly ground pepper to taste.

NUTRITIONAL VALUE per serving

Calories	162
Fat, total	10 g
Fat, saturated	2 g
Cholesterol	0 mg
Sodium	178 mg
Carbohydrate	18 g
Fiber	1 g
Protein	2 g
Calcium	86 mg
Iron	1 mg

Red Lentil Dosas

Makes 6 dosas (1 per serving)

Dosa is a flourless bread of southern India. More like pancakes, dosas are traditionally dipped into a curry or eaten with mango chutney.

Tips

Dosa batter should be the thickness of crêpe batter.

To test a skillet for the correct temperature (375°F/190°C), sprinkle a few drops of water on the hot surface. If the water bounces and dances across the pan, it is ready to use. If the water sizzles and evaporates, it is too hot. Adjust the heat if necessary to accommodate differences among cooking utensils and appliances.

◆ 10-inch (25 cm) cast-iron skillet, 2 inches (5 cm) deep, lightly greased

¾ cup	short-grain rice	175 mL
¼ cup	red lentils	50 mL
3 cups	warm water	750 mL
½ tsp	salt	2 mL
½ tsp	ground turmeric	2 mL
¼ tsp	freshly ground black pepper	1 mL
2 tbsp	chopped fresh cilantro	25 mL

1. In a large bowl, combine rice, lentils and water. Cover and let soak overnight at room temperature.

2. In a food processor fitted with a metal blade, purée rice and lentils with liquid until smooth. Spoon into a bowl, cover with plastic wrap and let stand in a warm place to ferment for 24 hours. Stir in salt, turmeric, pepper and cilantro.

3. Heat skillet over medium heat until hot. Add ¼ cup (50 mL) of batter. Using the rounded bottom of a large spoon, gently spread the batter in a circular motion to make a 6-inch (15 cm) diameter circle. Cook for 1½ to 2 minutes, or until set. Turn over and cook for about 1 minute, or until bottom is golden. Remove to a plate and cover with a lint-free towel to keep warm. Repeat with remaining batter, stacking the cooked dosas as you finish them and covering to keep warm.

Variation

Add ¼ cup (50 mL) grated coconut, 1 tbsp (15 mL) grated gingerroot and 1 finely chopped chili pepper to the batter just before cooking.

NUTRITIONAL VALUE per serving

Calories	116
Fat, total	0 g
Fat, saturated	0 g
Cholesterol	0 mg
Sodium	201 mg
Carbohydrate	25 g
Fiber	1 g
Protein	4 g
Calcium	12 mg
Iron	1 mg

Soda Bread

Makes 8 wedges (1 per serving)

Like the traditional hearth bread, this loaf features a crusty exterior and a soft, slightly tangy interior with a pronounced soda flavor. It's perfect with Irish stew or baked beans.

Tip

To make almond flour, see under Nut flour in the Technique Glossary, page 301.

* Preheat oven to 375°F (190°C)
* 8-inch (2 L) round baking pan, lightly greased

1 cup	fortified soy beverage, lactose-free milk or milk	250 mL
1 tbsp	freshly squeezed lemon juice	15 mL
2/3 cup	brown rice flour	150 mL
1/3 cup	almond flour	75 mL
1/3 cup	GF oat flour	75 mL
1/4 cup	tapioca starch	50 mL
1 tbsp	granulated sugar	15 mL
1 1/2 tsp	xanthan gum	7 mL
2 tsp	baking soda	10 mL
1 tsp	cream of tartar	5 mL
1/4 tsp	salt	1 mL
1/4 cup	lactose-free buttery spread or butter	50 mL

1. In a measuring cup or bowl, combine soy beverage and lemon juice; set aside for 5 minutes.

2. In a large bowl, combine brown rice flour, almond flour, oat flour, tapioca starch, sugar, xanthan gum, baking soda, cream of tartar and salt. Using a pastry blender or 2 knives, cut in buttery spread until mixture resembles coarse crumbs about the size of small peas. Add soy beverage mixture all at once, stirring with a fork to make a soft, slightly sticky dough.

3. Spoon dough into prepared pan. With a sharp knife, lightly score 1/8 inch (3 mm) deep into 8 wedges.

4. Bake in preheated oven for 20 to 25 minutes, or until a cake tester inserted in the center comes out clean. Let cool in pan on a rack for 5 minutes. Cut into wedges and serve hot.

Variation

For a fruited version, add 1 cup (250 mL) raisins, currants and/or chopped walnuts to the dry ingredients before adding the soy beverage mixture.

NUTRITIONAL VALUE per serving

Calories	127
Fat, total	5 g
Fat, saturated	1 g
Cholesterol	0 mg
Sodium	439 mg
Carbohydrate	18 g
Fiber	2 g
Protein	3 g
Calcium	49 mg
Iron	1 mg

Skillet Cornbread

Makes 10 to 12 wedges (1 per serving)

Our version of Johnny Cake (thought to be a corruption of "journey cake") is delicious served hot for lunch with a crisp salad.

Tip

For information on cleaning and seasoning a cast-iron skillet, see the Technique Glossary, page 299.

♦ Preheat oven to 400°F (200°C)
♦ 10-inch (25 cm) cast-iron skillet, 2 inches (5 cm) deep

1⅓ cups	fortified soy beverage, lactose-free milk or milk	325 mL
1 tbsp	cider vinegar	15 mL
1 cup	cornmeal	250 mL
	Vegetable oil for skillet	
¾ cup	soy flour	175 mL
¼ cup	tapioca starch	50 mL
¼ cup	granulated sugar	50 mL
1½ tsp	xanthan gum	7 mL
2 tsp	GF baking powder	10 mL
1 tsp	baking soda	5 mL
1 tsp	salt	5 mL
2	eggs	2
¼ cup	vegetable oil	50 mL

1. In a medium bowl, combine soy beverage, vinegar and cornmeal; set aside for 20 minutes.
2. Lightly brush sides of skillet with oil. Heat pan for 10 minutes in preheated oven.
3. In a bowl or large plastic bag, combine soy flour, tapioca starch, sugar, xanthan gum, baking powder, baking soda and salt. Mix well and set aside.
4. In a separate bowl, using an electric mixer, beat eggs and ¼ cup (50 mL) oil. Stir in soy beverage mixture. Add dry ingredients and mix just until combined.
5. Carefully spoon batter into hot skillet. Bake in preheated oven for 20 to 25 minutes, or until a cake tester inserted in the center comes out clean. Let cool in pan on a rack for 10 minutes. Cut into wedges and serve warm.

NUTRITIONAL VALUE per serving

Calories	149
Fat, total	6 g
Fat, saturated	1 g
Cholesterol	31 mg
Sodium	326 mg
Carbohydrate	19 g
Fiber	1 g
Protein	6 g
Calcium	90 mg
Iron	1 mg

Tip

To prevent a cast-iron skillet from rusting, set it on a warm stove element to dry completely before storing. Be careful: the handle gets hot.

To make this recipe egg-free

Omit eggs from recipe. Add 2 tsp (10 mL) powdered egg replacer with the dry ingredients and increase the soy beverage to 1⅔ cups (400 mL).

Variations

For a Maritime or New England version, add ¼ cup (50 mL) molasses with the eggs and increase the cornmeal to 1¼ cups (300 mL).

For a spicier version, add a 4-oz (113 g) can of chopped green chili peppers, well drained, with the eggs.

Add 6 slices of GF bacon, cooked crisp and crumbled, with the dry ingredients.

For a dessert cornbread, increase the sugar to ½ cup (125 mL) and serve warm, drizzled with maple syrup.

Bacon Dijon Muffins or Loaf

A hint of sweet mustard contrasts with the savory, smoky bacon to give these muffins or loaf slices a unique flavor.

Tip

For crisp texture, microwave the bacon on High for 6 to 8 minutes, or until crisp. Drain well on paper towels.

NUTRITIONAL VALUE per serving	
Calories	171
Fat, total	7 g
Fat, saturated	1 g
Cholesterol	23 mg
Sodium	224 mg
Carbohydrate	25 g
Fiber	2 g
Protein	5 g
Calcium	82 mg
Iron	1 mg

♦ 12-cup muffin tin or 9- by 5-inch (2 L) loaf pan, lightly greased

1 cup	sorghum flour	250 mL
⅓ cup	quinoa flour	75 mL
⅓ cup	potato starch	75 mL
1½ tsp	xanthan gum	7 mL
1 tbsp	GF baking powder	15 mL
¼ tsp	salt	1 mL
2 tsp	dried sage	10 mL
¼ tsp	dry mustard	1 mL
1	egg	1
1 cup	water	250 mL
2 tbsp	vegetable oil	25 mL
¼ cup	liquid honey	50 mL
2 tbsp	Dijon mustard	25 mL
8	slices GF bacon, cooked crisp and crumbled	8

1. In a large bowl or plastic bag, combine sorghum flour, quinoa flour, potato starch, xanthan gum, baking powder, salt, sage and dry mustard. Mix well and set aside.

2. In a separate bowl, using an electric mixer, beat egg, water, oil, honey and Dijon mustard until combined. Add dry ingredients and mix just until combined. Stir in bacon.

For Muffins

3. Spoon batter evenly into each of 10 cups of prepared muffin tin. Let stand for 30 minutes. Meanwhile, preheat oven to 350°F (180°C). Bake for 18 to 20 minutes, or until firm to the touch. Remove from pan immediately and let cool completely on a rack.

For a Loaf

3. Spoon batter into prepared loaf pan. Let stand for 30 minutes. Meanwhile, preheat oven to 350°F (180°C). Bake for 45 to 55 minutes, or until a cake tester inserted in the center comes out clean. Let cool in pan on a rack for 10 minutes. Remove from pan and let cool completely on rack.

Tips

Fill the empty muffin cups half full of water.

Only fill the muffin cups half full, as these muffins rise to be regular size upon baking.

To make this recipe egg-free

Omit egg from recipe. Add 2 tsp (10 mL) powdered egg replacer with the dry ingredients and increase the water to $1\frac{1}{3}$ cups (325 mL). Increase baking time by 2 to 3 minutes for muffins or loaf.

Variations

Substitute another flavor of mustard for the Dijon, such as tarragon or green peppercorn. Be sure to check the ingredient list for gluten.

Make 12 slightly smaller muffins or 18 mini muffins.

Apricot Almond Muffins or Loaf

Perfect to pack for office or school lunches, these muffins or loaf slices are moist but not too sweet, with the sunny goodness of orange and apricot and the tang of yogurt.

Tip

Snip dried apricots into ¼-inch (0.5 cm) pieces with sharp scissors. Dip blades into hot water when they become sticky.

◆ 12-cup muffin tin or 9- by 5-inch (2 L) loaf pan, lightly greased

1 cup	amaranth flour	250 mL
½ cup	sorghum flour	125 mL
⅓ cup	almond flour	75 mL
¼ cup	tapioca starch	50 mL
½ cup	granulated sugar	125 mL
1½ tsp	xanthan gum	7 mL
1 tbsp	GF baking powder	15 mL
½ tsp	baking soda	2 mL
½ tsp	salt	2 mL
1 tsp	ground nutmeg	5 mL
2	eggs	2
2 tbsp	grated orange zest	25 mL
2 tbsp	vegetable oil	25 mL
1¼ cups	lactose-free plain yogurt or plain yogurt	300 mL
1 cup	snipped dried apricots	250 mL
1 cup	toasted slivered almonds	250 mL

1. In a large bowl or plastic bag, combine amaranth flour, sorghum flour, almond flour, tapioca starch, sugar, xanthan gum, baking powder, baking soda, salt and nutmeg. Mix well and set aside.

2. In a separate bowl, using an electric mixer, beat eggs, orange zest, oil and yogurt until combined. Add dry ingredients and mix just until combined. Stir in apricots and almonds.

For Muffins

3. Spoon batter evenly into each cup of prepared muffin tin. Let stand for 30 minutes. Meanwhile, preheat oven to 350°F (180°C). Bake for 18 to 20 minutes, or until firm to the touch. Remove from pan immediately and let cool completely on a rack.

NUTRITIONAL VALUE per serving	
Calories	265
Fat, total	12 g
Fat, saturated	1 g
Cholesterol	31 mg
Sodium	152 mg
Carbohydrate	34 g
Fiber	4 g
Protein	8 g
Calcium	121 mg
Iron	4 mg

Tip

See the Technique Glossary, page 301, for instructions on toasting nuts.

For a Loaf

3. Spoon batter into prepared loaf pan. Let stand for 30 minutes. Meanwhile, preheat oven to 350°F (180°C). Bake for 55 to 65 minutes, or until a cake tester inserted in the center comes out clean. Let cool in pan on a rack for 10 minutes. Remove from pan and let cool completely on rack.

To make this recipe egg-free
Omit eggs from recipe. Add 2 tbsp (25 mL) powdered egg replacer with the dry ingredients and $1/3$ cup (75 mL) warm water with the yogurt. Increase baking time by 2 to 3 minutes for muffins or loaf.

Variation

Substitute ground cinnamon or $1/2$ tsp (2 mL) cloves for the nutmeg.

Blueberry Flax Muffins or Loaf

Makes 12 muffins or 12 slices (1 per serving)

We are all conscious of the antioxidant properties of blueberries and the health benefits of flax. We've combined them for you in this nutritious recipe.

Tip

For information on cracking flaxseed, see the Technique Glossary, page 300.

If using frozen blueberries, thaw and gently pat dry with paper towels.

◆ *12-cup muffin tin or 9- by 5-inch (2 L) loaf pan, lightly greased*

1 cup	sorghum flour	250 mL
⅓ cup	quinoa flour	75 mL
⅓ cup	flax flour	75 mL
¼ cup	tapioca starch	50 mL
1½ tsp	xanthan gum	7 mL
1 tbsp	GF baking powder	15 mL
½ tsp	salt	2 mL
¼ cup	flaxseed, cracked	50 mL
1	egg	1
2 tbsp	grated orange zest	25 mL
1 cup	freshly squeezed orange juice	250 mL
2 tbsp	vegetable oil	25 mL
½ cup	pure maple syrup	125 mL
1 cup	fresh or frozen blueberries, thawed	250 mL

1. In a large bowl or plastic bag, combine sorghum flour, quinoa flour, flax flour, tapioca starch, xanthan gum, baking powder, salt and flaxseed. Mix well and set aside.

2. In a separate bowl, using an electric mixer, beat egg, orange zest, orange juice, oil and maple syrup until combined. Add dry ingredients and mix just until combined. Carefully fold in blueberries.

For Muffins

3. Spoon batter evenly into each cup of prepared muffin tin. Let stand for 30 minutes. Meanwhile, preheat oven to 350°F (180°C). Bake for 22 to 25 minutes, or until firm to the touch. Remove from pan immediately and let cool completely on a rack.

NUTRITIONAL VALUE per serving	
Calories	173
Fat, total	6 g
Fat, saturated	1 g
Cholesterol	16 mg
Sodium	109 mg
Carbohydrate	29 g
Fiber	4 g
Protein	10 g
Calcium	91 mg
Iron	2 mg

Tip

If using frozen blueberries, thaw and gently pat dry with paper towels.

For a Loaf

3. Spoon batter into prepared loaf pan. Let stand for 30 minutes. Meanwhile, preheat oven to 350°F (180°C). Bake for 55 to 65 minutes, or until a cake tester inserted in the center comes out clean. Let cool in pan on a rack for 10 minutes. Remove from pan and let cool completely on rack.

To make this recipe egg-free
Omit egg from recipe. Combine an additional 2 tbsp (25 mL) flax flour or ground flaxseed with ¼ cup (50 mL) warm water. Let stand for 5 minutes. Add with liquids. Increase baking time by 2 to 3 minutes for muffins or loaf.

Variations

Substitute ground flaxseed for the flax flour.

Substitute pancake syrup for the maple syrup.

Chocolate–Chocolate Chip Muffins or Loaf

Makes 12 muffins or 12 slices (1 per serving)

This recipe brings out the kid in all of us. Who can resist chocolate, the original comfort food? These taste more like brownies than muffins.

Tip

If muffins stick to the pan, let cool for 2 to 3 minutes, then try again to remove them.

◆ 12-cup muffin tin or 9- by 5-inch (2 L) loaf pan, lightly greased

¾ cup	sorghum flour	175 mL
⅓ cup	quinoa flour	75 mL
¼ cup	tapioca starch	50 mL
½ cup	granulated sugar	125 mL
1 tsp	xanthan gum	5 mL
2 tsp	GF baking powder	10 mL
1 tsp	baking soda	5 mL
¼ tsp	salt	1 mL
¼ cup	unsweetened cocoa powder, sifted	50 mL
2	eggs	2
1 cup	lactose-free sour cream or sour cream	250 mL
¼ cup	vegetable oil	50 mL
⅔ cup	lactose-free chocolate chips or chocolate chips	150 mL

1. In a large bowl or plastic bag, combine sorghum flour, quinoa flour, tapioca starch, sugar, xanthan gum, baking powder, baking soda, salt and cocoa. Mix well and set aside.

2. In a separate bowl, using an electric mixer, beat eggs, sour cream and oil until combined. Add dry ingredients and mix just until combined. Stir in chocolate chips.

For Muffins

3. Spoon batter evenly into each cup of prepared muffin tin. Let stand for 30 minutes. Meanwhile, preheat oven to 350°F (180°C). Bake for 18 to 20 minutes, or until firm to the touch. Remove from pan immediately and let cool completely on a rack.

NUTRITIONAL VALUE per serving

Calories	216
Fat, total	11 g
Fat, saturated	3 g
Cholesterol	31 mg
Sodium	249 mg
Carbohydrate	27 g
Fiber	2 g
Protein	4 g
Calcium	47 mg
Iron	2 mg

Tip

Use an ice cream scoop to portion an even amount of batter into each muffin cup. These are large muffins.

For a Loaf

3. Spoon batter into prepared loaf pan. Let stand for 30 minutes. Meanwhile, preheat oven to 350°F (180°C). Bake for 55 to 65 minutes, or until a cake tester inserted in the center comes out clean. Let cool in pan on a rack for 10 minutes. Remove from pan and let cool completely on rack.

To make this recipe egg-free

Omit eggs from recipe. Add 1 tbsp (15 mL) powdered egg replacer with the dry ingredients and ⅓ cup (75 mL) water with the liquids. Increase baking time by 2 to 3 minutes for muffins or loaf.

Variations

If quinoa flour is not available, substitute an equal amount of brown rice flour.

Substitute jumbo or mini chocolate chips — just be sure they are lactose-free, if necessary.

Date Nut Muffins or Loaf

**Makes 12 muffins
or 12 slices
(1 per serving)**

Dates and nuts are a
classic combination,
but we always think of
them in terms of this
traditional muffin or loaf.
Its moist, dark, sweet
flavor is full of comfort
and fond memories.

Tip

If you purchase chopped
instead of whole dates, be
sure to check for gluten.

◆ 12-cup muffin tin or 9- by 5-inch (2 L) loaf pan, lightly
  greased

1 cup	coarsely chopped dates	250 mL
½ cup	chopped walnuts	125 mL
3 tbsp	shortening or vegetable oil	45 mL
2 tsp	baking soda	10 mL
½ tsp	salt	2 mL
1 cup	boiling water	250 mL
¾ cup	sorghum flour	175 mL
⅔ cup	whole bean flour	150 mL
¼ cup	tapioca starch	50 mL
¾ cup	granulated sugar	175 mL
1½ tsp	xanthan gum	7 mL
2	eggs	2
1 tsp	vanilla	5 mL

1. In a medium bowl, combine dates, walnuts,
   shortening, baking soda and salt. Pour in boiling
   water and set aside for 20 minutes.

2. In a large bowl or plastic bag, combine sorghum flour,
   whole bean flour, tapioca starch, sugar and xanthan
   gum. Mix well and set aside.

3. In a separate bowl, using an electric mixer, beat eggs
   and vanilla until combined. Stir in date mixture. Add
   dry ingredients and mix just until combined.

For Muffins

3. Spoon batter evenly into each cup of prepared muffin
   tin. Let stand for 30 minutes. Meanwhile, preheat
   oven to 350°F (180°C). Bake for 18 to 20 minutes, or
   until firm to the touch. Remove from pan immediately
   and let cool completely on a rack.

**NUTRITIONAL VALUE
per serving**

Calories	214
Fat, total	8 g
Fat, saturated	1 g
Cholesterol	31 mg
Sodium	319 mg
Carbohydrate	35 g
Fiber	3 g
Protein	4 g
Calcium	21 mg
Iron	1 mg

We use kitchen shears to snip whole dates into eighths, dipping shears in hot water as they become sticky. If you purchase chopped dates, check for wheat starch in the coating.

For a Loaf

3. Spoon batter into prepared loaf pan. Let stand for 30 minutes. Meanwhile, preheat oven to 350°F (180°C). Bake for 55 to 65 minutes, or until a cake tester inserted in the center comes out clean. Let cool in pan on a rack for 10 minutes. Remove from pan and let cool completely on rack.

To make this recipe egg-free

Omit eggs from recipe. Combine $1/4$ cup (50 mL) flax flour or ground flaxseed with $1/3$ cup (75 mL) warm water. Let stand for 5 minutes. Add with vanilla. Increase baking time by 2 to 3 minutes for muffins or loaf.

Variation

Replace half the dates with the same quantity of figs.

Fruited Barm Brack Muffins or Loaf

Makes 12 muffins or 12 slices (1 per serving)

Barm brack — which means "yeast bread" in Gaelic, although it is not always made with yeast — is an Irish bread with raisins or currants and candied fruit peel. Try our fruited version, made with tea, apricots and cranberries. Perfect with an entrée or dessert.

Tip

Powdered ice tea mixes are too sweet and too strongly flavored with lemon to be substituted for the tea in this recipe.

◆ 12-cup muffin tin or 9- by 5-inch (2 L) loaf pan, lightly greased

1¼ cups	amaranth flour	300 mL
⅓ cup	sorghum flour	75 mL
¼ cup	tapioca starch	50 mL
½ cup	packed brown sugar	125 mL
1½ tsp	xanthan gum	7 mL
1 tbsp	GF baking powder	15 mL
1 tsp	baking soda	5 mL
½ tsp	salt	2 mL
1½ tsp	ground cinnamon	7 mL
1 tsp	ground nutmeg	5 mL
1	egg	1
1 cup	strong brewed black tea, at room temperature	250 mL
3 tbsp	vegetable oil	45 mL
½ cup	snipped dried apricots	125 mL
½ cup	currants	125 mL
½ cup	dried cranberries	125 mL

1. In a large bowl or plastic bag, combine amaranth flour, sorghum flour, tapioca starch, brown sugar, xanthan gum, baking powder, baking soda, salt, cinnamon and nutmeg. Mix well and set aside.

2. In a separate bowl, using an electric mixer, beat egg, tea and oil until combined. Add dry ingredients and mix just until combined. Stir in apricots, currants and cranberries.

For Muffins

3. Spoon batter evenly into each cup of prepared muffin tin. Let stand for 30 minutes. Meanwhile, preheat oven to 350°F (180°C). Bake for 18 to 20 minutes, or until firm to the touch. Remove from pan immediately and let cool completely on a rack.

NUTRITIONAL VALUE per serving	
Calories	174
Fat, total	5 g
Fat, saturated	0 g
Cholesterol	16 mg
Sodium	214 mg
Carbohydrate	31 g
Fiber	2 g
Protein	3 g
Calcium	91 mg
Iron	4 mg

We allow our tea to steep longer than usual to make it extra strong for this recipe.

For a Loaf

3. Spoon batter into prepared loaf pan. Let stand for 30 minutes. Meanwhile, preheat oven to 350°F (180°C). Bake for 55 to 65 minutes, or until a cake tester inserted in the center comes out clean. Let cool in pan on a rack for 10 minutes. Remove from pan and let cool completely on rack.

To make this recipe egg-free
Omit egg from recipe. Add 2 tsp (10 mL) powdered egg replacer with the dry ingredients and $1/4$ cup (50 mL) water with the liquids. Increase baking time by 2 to 3 minutes for muffins or loaf.

Variation
Try replacing one or more of the fruits with an equal quantity of snipped dried cherries, dried apples or dates.

Golden Harvest Muffins or Loaf

Makes 12 muffins or 12 slices (1 per serving)

The warm color of these muffins or loaf slices reminds us of an autumn wheat field ready for harvest.

Tip

Microwave the sweet potato as you would a regular baking potato, until fork-tender. (Cooking time will depend on the size of the potato.) Peel, then mash when cool enough to handle.

◆ 12-cup muffin tin or 9- by 5-inch (2 L) loaf pan, lightly greased

⅔ cup	amaranth flour	150 mL
½ cup	pea flour	125 mL
½ cup	cornmeal	125 mL
¼ cup	packed brown sugar	50 mL
1½ tsp	xanthan gum	7 mL
1 tbsp	GF baking powder	15 mL
½ tsp	salt	2 mL
1	egg	1
1 tbsp	grated orange zest	15 mL
½ cup	freshly squeezed orange juice	125 mL
¼ cup	vegetable oil	50 mL
1 cup	mashed cooked sweet potato, at room temperature (see tip, at left)	250 mL
¼ cup	pure maple syrup	50 mL
¾ cup	chopped dried apricots	175 mL

1. In a large bowl or plastic bag, combine amaranth flour, pea flour, cornmeal, brown sugar, xanthan gum, baking powder and salt. Mix well and set aside.

2. In a separate bowl, using an electric mixer, beat egg, orange zest, orange juice and oil until combined. Add sweet potato and maple syrup while mixing. Add dry ingredients and mix just until combined. Stir in apricots.

For Muffins

3. Spoon batter evenly into each cup of prepared muffin tin. Let stand for 30 minutes. Meanwhile, preheat oven to 350°F (180°C). Bake for 18 to 20 minutes, or until firm to the touch. Remove from pan immediately and let cool completely on a rack.

NUTRITIONAL VALUE per serving	
Calories	199
Fat, total	6 g
Fat, saturated	1 g
Cholesterol	16 mg
Sodium	111 mg
Carbohydrate	35 g
Fiber	3 g
Protein	4 g
Calcium	88 mg
Iron	3 mg

Wet pea flour has a strong
odor that disappears
when it is baked.

For a Loaf

3. Spoon batter into prepared loaf pan. Let stand for
30 minutes. Meanwhile, preheat oven to 350°F
(180°C). Bake for 55 to 65 minutes, or until a cake
tester inserted in the center comes out clean. Let cool
in pan on a rack for 10 minutes. Remove from pan
and let cool completely on rack.

To make this recipe egg-free
Omit egg from recipe. Add 1 tsp (5 mL) powdered
egg replacer with the dry ingredients and 2 tbsp
(25 mL) water with the liquid. Increase baking
time by 2 to 3 minutes for muffins or loaf.

Variations

Substitute canned sweet potatoes or yams, well
drained, for the fresh.

Substitute ¼ cup (50 mL) currants for an equal
amount of chopped apricots.

Nutty Mocha Java Muffins or Loaf

Makes 12 muffins or 12 slices (1 per serving)

Here's the ultimate dessert combo — double coffee, chocolate, orange and hazelnuts — all in one delectable treat!

Tip

Don't chop the hazelnuts too finely or you'll lose the crunchy texture.

♦ 12-cup muffin tin or 9- by 5-inch (2 L) loaf pan, lightly greased

1 cup	sorghum flour	250 mL
⅓ cup	whole bean flour	75 mL
¼ cup	tapioca starch	50 mL
¼ cup	packed brown sugar	50 mL
1½ tsp	xanthan gum	7 mL
1 tbsp	GF baking powder	15 mL
½ tsp	salt	2 mL
3 tbsp	unsweetened cocoa powder, sifted	45 mL
1	egg	1
1 tbsp	grated orange zest	15 mL
1 cup	strong brewed coffee, at room temperature	250 mL
1 tbsp	coffee-flavored liqueur	15 mL
¼ cup	vegetable oil	50 mL
½ cup	corn syrup	125 mL
¾ cup	coarsely chopped hazelnuts	175 mL

1. In a large bowl or plastic bag, combine sorghum flour, whole bean flour, tapioca starch, brown sugar, xanthan gum, baking powder, salt and cocoa. Mix well and set aside.

2. In a separate bowl, using an electric mixer, beat egg, orange zest, coffee, liqueur and oil until combined. Add corn syrup while mixing. Add dry ingredients and mix just until combined. Stir in hazelnuts.

For Muffins

3. Spoon batter evenly into each cup of prepared muffin tin. Let stand for 30 minutes. Meanwhile, preheat oven to 350°F (180°C). Bake for 18 to 20 minutes, or until firm to the touch. Remove from pan immediately and let cool completely on a rack.

NUTRITIONAL VALUE per serving

Calories	216
Fat, total	10 g
Fat, saturated	1 g
Cholesterol	16 mg
Sodium	122 mg
Carbohydrate	30 g
Fiber	2 g
Protein	3 g
Calcium	80 mg
Iron	2 mg

Tip

Use any coffee-flavored liqueur, such as Tia Maria.

For a Loaf

3. Spoon batter into prepared loaf pan. Let stand for 30 minutes. Meanwhile, preheat oven to 350°F (180°C). Bake for 55 to 65 minutes, or until a cake tester inserted in the center comes out clean. Let cool in pan on a rack for 10 minutes. Remove from pan and let cool completely on rack.

> **To make this recipe egg-free**
> Omit egg from recipe. Combine 2 tbsp (25 mL) flax flour or ground flaxseed with $\frac{1}{4}$ cup (50 mL) warm water. Let stand for 5 minutes. Add with liquid ingredients. Increase baking time by 2 to 3 minutes for muffins or loaf.

Variation

In place of liqueur, substitute thawed frozen orange juice concentrate.

Oatmeal Rhubarb Muffins or Loaf

Makes 12 muffins or 12 slices (1 per serving)

These are more like cupcakes than muffins or loaf slices — so tangy, moist and nutritious you'll go back for seconds.

Tip

You can use fresh or frozen rhubarb. If using frozen, partially thaw in the microwave before chopping finely. Drain well, then pat dry with paper towels.

♦ *12-cup muffin tin or 9- by 5-inch (2 L) loaf pan, lightly greased*

¾ cup	sorghum flour	175 mL
⅔ cup	GF oat flour	150 mL
⅓ cup	GF oats	75 mL
¼ cup	tapioca starch	50 mL
¾ cup	packed brown sugar	175 mL
1½ tsp	xanthan gum	7 mL
1 tsp	baking soda	5 mL
½ tsp	salt	2 mL
1 tsp	ground cinnamon	5 mL
1	egg	1
1 tbsp	grated lemon zest	15 mL
1 tbsp	freshly squeezed lemon juice	15 mL
¼ cup	vegetable oil	50 mL
1 cup	fortified soy beverage, lactose-free milk or milk	250 mL
1½ cups	finely chopped rhubarb	375 mL

1. In a large bowl or plastic bag, combine sorghum flour, oat flour, oats, tapioca starch, brown sugar, xanthan gum, baking soda, salt and cinnamon. Mix well and set aside.

2. In a separate bowl, using an electric mixer, beat egg, lemon zest, lemon juice, oil and soy beverage until combined. Add dry ingredients and mix just until combined. Stir in rhubarb.

For Muffins

3. Spoon batter evenly into each cup of prepared muffin tin. Let stand for 30 minutes. Meanwhile, preheat oven to 350°F (180°C). Bake for 20 to 23 minutes, or until firm to the touch. Remove from pan immediately and let cool completely on a rack.

NUTRITIONAL VALUE per serving

Calories	174
Fat, total	6 g
Fat, saturated	1 g
Cholesterol	16 mg
Sodium	224 mg
Carbohydrate	29 g
Fiber	2 g
Protein	3 g
Calcium	62 mg
Iron	1 mg

Tip

For information on GF oats and oat flour, see pages 37–39.

For a Loaf

3. Spoon batter into prepared loaf pan. Let stand for 30 minutes. Meanwhile, preheat oven to 350°F (180°C). Bake for 60 to 70 minutes, or until a cake tester inserted in the center comes out clean. Let cool in pan on a rack for 10 minutes. Remove from pan and let cool completely on rack.

> **To make this recipe egg-free**
> Omit egg from recipe. Combine 2 tbsp (25 mL) flax flour or ground flaxseed with 2 tbsp (25 mL) warm water. Let stand for 5 minutes. Add with liquid ingredients. Increase baking time by 2 to 3 minutes for muffins or loaf.

Variation

Season with ½ tsp (2 mL) ground ginger instead of the cinnamon. Add ½ cup (125 mL) chopped pecans with the rhubarb for added crunch.

Rhubarb Orange Muffins or Loaf

Makes 12 muffins or 12 slices (1 per serving)

Looking for a new way to enjoy the first fruit of the spring harvest? Try this soft, slightly sweet muffin or loaf.

Tip

When using frozen rhubarb, it is easier to chop while still partially frozen. The rhubarb must be finely chopped; otherwise, the finished muffin will be crumbly.

♦ *12-cup muffin tin or 9- by 5-inch (2 L) loaf pan, lightly greased*

1¾ cups	finely chopped rhubarb	425 mL
⅓ cup	granulated sugar	75 mL
1⅓ cups	sorghum flour	325 mL
⅓ cup	quinoa flour	75 mL
⅓ cup	potato starch	75 mL
1½ tsp	xanthan gum	7 mL
1 tbsp	GF baking powder	15 mL
1 tsp	baking soda	5 mL
½ tsp	salt	2 mL
1	egg	1
2 tbsp	grated orange zest	25 mL
⅔ cup	freshly squeezed orange juice	150 mL
3 tbsp	vegetable oil	45 mL
1 tsp	vanilla	5 mL
½ cup	chopped walnuts	125 mL

1. In a medium bowl, combine rhubarb and sugar. Mix well and set aside for 10 minutes.

2. In a large bowl or plastic bag, combine sorghum flour, quinoa flour, potato starch, xanthan gum, baking powder, baking soda and salt. Mix well and set aside.

3. In a separate bowl, using an electric mixer, beat egg, orange zest, orange juice, oil and vanilla until combined. Stir in rhubarb mixture. Add dry ingredients and mix just until combined. Stir in walnuts.

For Muffins

3. Spoon batter evenly into each cup of prepared muffin tin. Let stand for 30 minutes. Meanwhile, preheat oven to 350°F (180°C). Bake for 18 to 20 minutes, or until firm to the touch. Remove from pan immediately and let cool completely on a rack.

NUTRITIONAL VALUE per serving

Calories	183
Fat, total	8 g
Fat, saturated	1 g
Cholesterol	16 mg
Sodium	210 mg
Carbohydrate	27 g
Fiber	3 g
Protein	4 g
Calcium	110 mg
Iron	1 mg

Tip

One orange yields about 1½ tbsp (22 mL) of zest and ⅓ to ½ cup (75 to 125 mL) of juice. To get the most juice out of your oranges, bring them to room temperature, then roll them on the counter or between your hands. It's worth the time and effort it takes to zest fresh oranges and squeeze fresh juice. Freeze any extra zest and juice for next time.

For a Loaf

3. Spoon batter into prepared loaf pan. Let stand for 30 minutes. Meanwhile, preheat oven to 350°F (180°C). Bake for 55 to 65 minutes, or until a cake tester inserted in the center comes out clean. Let cool in pan on a rack for 10 minutes. Remove from pan and let cool completely on rack.

> **To make this recipe egg-free**
> Omit eggs from recipe. Combine 2 tbsp (25 mL) flax flour or ground flaxseed with ¼ cup (50 mL) warm water. Let stand for 5 minutes. Add with liquid ingredients. Increase baking time by 2 to 3 minutes for muffins or loaf.

Variation

Substitute pecans or ¼ cup (50 mL) green pumpkin seeds for the walnuts.

Sun-Dried Tomato Rice Muffins or Loaf

Makes 12 muffins or 12 slices (1 per serving)

Prefer a savory muffin or loaf to a sweet one? The spicy tomato-basil flavor in this recipe complements any soup or salad.

Tips

Oil-packed sun-dried tomatoes are not suited to this recipe. For the best results, look for soft, pliable dry-packed sun-dried tomatoes.

See "Cooking Rice," page 46, for instructions on cooking wild rice.

When cooking wild rice, do not add salt to the water.

NUTRITIONAL VALUE per serving	
Calories	132
Fat, total	4 g
Fat, saturated	1 g
Cholesterol	31 mg
Sodium	110 mg
Carbohydrate	22 g
Fiber	2 g
Protein	4 g
Calcium	75 mg
Iron	2 mg

♦ 12-cup muffin tin or 9- by 5-inch (2 L) loaf pan, lightly greased

1 cup	sorghum flour	250 mL
⅓ cup	quinoa flour	75 mL
⅓ cup	tapioca starch	75 mL
3 tbsp	packed brown sugar	45 mL
1½ tsp	xanthan gum	7 mL
1 tbsp	GF baking powder	15 mL
¼ tsp	salt	1 mL
1 tbsp	dried basil	15 mL
2	eggs	2
2 tbsp	extra-virgin olive oil	25 mL
1 cup	water	250 mL
1 cup	cooked wild rice	250 mL
½ cup	snipped dry-packed sun-dried tomatoes	125 mL

1. In a large bowl or plastic bag, combine sorghum flour, quinoa flour, tapioca starch, brown sugar, xanthan gum, baking powder, salt and basil. Mix well and set aside.

2. In a separate bowl, using an electric mixer, beat eggs, oil and water until combined. Add dry ingredients and mix just until combined. Stir in wild rice and sun-dried tomatoes.

For Muffins

3. Spoon batter evenly into each cup of prepared muffin tin. Let stand for 30 minutes. Meanwhile, preheat oven to 350°F (180°C). Bake for 20 to 23 minutes, or until firm to the touch. Remove from pan immediately and let cool completely on a rack.

Cook extra wild rice for dinner and refrigerate overnight to use in this recipe.

For a Loaf

3. Spoon batter into prepared loaf pan. Let stand for 30 minutes. Meanwhile, preheat oven to 350°F (180°C). Bake for 60 to 70 minutes, or until a cake tester inserted in the center comes out clean. Let cool in pan on a rack for 10 minutes. Remove from pan and let cool completely on rack.

To make this recipe egg-free
Omit eggs from recipe. Combine $\frac{1}{4}$ cup (50 mL) flax flour or ground flaxseed with $\frac{1}{3}$ cup (75 mL) warm water. Let stand for 5 minutes. Add with liquid ingredients. Increase baking time by 2 to 3 minutes for muffins or loaf.

Variation
Substitute $\frac{1}{4}$ cup (50 mL) frozen orange juice concentrate, thawed, for the same amount of water.

Toasted Walnut Pear Muffins or Loaf

Makes 12 muffins or 12 slices (1 per serving)

These high-fiber muffins or loaf slices with a delicate pear flavor are the perfect midmorning snack.

Tip

See the Technique Glossary, page 301, for instructions on toasting nuts.

♦ *12-cup muffin tin or 9- by 5-inch (2 L) loaf pan, lightly greased*

1¼ cups	sorghum flour	300 mL
⅔ cup	amaranth flour	150 mL
¼ cup	tapioca starch	50 mL
1½ tsp	xanthan gum	7 mL
1 tbsp	GF baking powder	15 mL
½ tsp	salt	2 mL
2	eggs	2
2 tbsp	walnut oil	25 mL
¾ cup	water	175 mL
¼ cup	pure maple syrup	50 mL
1 cup	toasted chopped walnuts	250 mL
⅓ cup	diced drained canned pears	75 mL

1. In a large bowl or plastic bag, combine sorghum flour, amaranth flour, tapioca starch, xanthan gum, baking powder and salt. Mix well and set aside.

2. In a separate bowl, using an electric mixer, beat eggs, walnut oil, water and syrup until combined. Add dry ingredients and mix just until combined. Stir in walnuts and pears.

For Muffins

3. Spoon batter evenly into each cup of prepared muffin tin. Let stand for 30 minutes. Meanwhile, preheat oven to 350°F (180°C). Bake for 20 to 23 minutes, or until firm to the touch. Remove from pan immediately and let cool completely on a rack.

NUTRITIONAL VALUE per serving

Calories	203
Fat, total	10 g
Fat, saturated	1 g
Cholesterol	31 mg
Sodium	109 mg
Carbohydrate	25 g
Fiber	3 g
Protein	5 g
Calcium	87 mg
Iron	3 mg

Tip

One 5-oz (142 mL) can of diced pears, drained, yields $\frac{1}{3}$ cup (75 mL) fruit.

For a Loaf

3. Spoon batter into prepared loaf pan. Let stand for 30 minutes. Meanwhile, preheat oven to 350°F (180°C). Bake for 60 to 70 minutes, or until a cake tester inserted in the center comes out clean. Let cool in pan on a rack for 10 minutes. Remove from pan and let cool completely on rack.

To make this recipe egg-free
Omit eggs from recipe. Combine $\frac{1}{4}$ cup (50 mL) flax flour or ground flaxseed with $\frac{1}{2}$ cup (125 mL) warm water. Let stand for 5 minutes. Add with liquid ingredients. Increase baking time by 2 to 3 minutes for muffins or loaf.

Variation

Replace the walnut oil with vegetable oil.

Wild Rice Cranberry Muffins or Loaf

The combination of wild rice and cranberries gives these muffins or loaf slices an interesting color and a lovely moist texture. They are sure to earn you compliments from both your celiac and non-celiac friends!

Tip

See "Cooking Rice," page 46, for instructions on cooking wild rice.

♦ 12-cup muffin tin or 9- by 5-inch (2 L) loaf pan, lightly greased

1 cup	amaranth flour	250 mL
1/3 cup	brown rice flour	75 mL
1/4 cup	tapioca starch	50 mL
1 1/2 tsp	xanthan gum	7 mL
1 tbsp	GF baking powder	15 mL
1 tsp	salt	5 mL
1 1/2 tsp	celery seeds	7 mL
1/4 tsp	freshly ground black pepper	1 mL
2	eggs	2
2 tbsp	extra-virgin olive oil	25 mL
3/4 cup	water	175 mL
1/4 cup	frozen orange juice concentrate, thawed	50 mL
1/4 cup	liquid honey	50 mL
1 cup	dried cranberries	250 mL
1 cup	cooked wild rice	250 mL
1/2 cup	pine nuts	125 mL

1. In a large bowl or plastic bag, combine amaranth flour, brown rice flour, tapioca starch, xanthan gum, baking powder, salt, celery seeds and pepper. Mix well and set aside.

2. In a separate bowl, using an electric mixer, beat eggs, oil, water and orange juice concentrate until combined. Add honey while mixing. Add dry ingredients and mix just until combined. Stir in cranberries, wild rice and pine nuts.

For Muffins

3. Spoon batter evenly into each cup of prepared muffin tin. Let stand for 30 minutes. Meanwhile, preheat oven to 350°F (180°C). Bake for 20 to 23 minutes, or until firm to the touch. Remove from pan immediately and let cool completely on a rack.

NUTRITIONAL VALUE per serving	
Calories	205
Fat, total	7 g
Fat, saturated	1 g
Cholesterol	31 mg
Sodium	207 mg
Carbohydrate	32 g
Fiber	1 g
Protein	5 g
Calcium	82 mg
Iron	4 mg

Tip

When cooking wild rice, do not add salt to the water.

For a Loaf

3. Spoon batter into prepared loaf pan. Let stand for 30 minutes. Meanwhile, preheat oven to 350°F (180°C). Bake for 60 to 70 minutes, or until a cake tester inserted in the center comes out clean. Let cool in pan on a rack for 10 minutes. Remove from pan and let cool completely on rack.

To make this recipe egg-free
Omit eggs from recipe. Combine $1/4$ cup (50 mL) flax flour or ground flaxseed with $1/2$ cup (125 mL) warm water. Let stand 5 minutes. Add with liquid ingredients. Increase baking time by 2 to 3 minutes for muffins or loaf.

Variation

Substitute unsalted sunflower seeds, soy nuts or chopped peanuts for the pine nuts.

Working with Muffin Mix

- Stir the mix before spooning very lightly into the dry measures when dividing into portions in Step 2 of method. Do not pack.
- Be sure to divide Make-Your-Own Muffin Mix (page 165) into 12 equal portions and Small-Batch Make-Your-Own Muffin Mix (page 166) into 3 equal portions before using to make up an individual recipe. Depending on how much air you incorporate into the mix and the texture of the individual gluten-free flours, the total volume of the mix can vary slightly. The important thing is to make equal portions.
- Label and date packages before storing. We add the page number of the recipe to the label as a quick reference.
- Let warm to room temperature and mix well before using.
- If you prefer to make a dozen muffins at a time, divide the mix into 6 portions of approximately 2½ cups (625 mL) and double all the ingredients listed in the individual muffin recipes.

Make-Your-Own Muffin Mix

Makes about 15 cups (3.75 L), or enough for 12 batches of 6 muffins each (1 muffin per serving)

When schedules are rushed, busy cooks often look for ways to shave time off the preparation of quick breads. Stock your freezer with mixes you prepare yourself. These do-it-yourself blends not only save minutes, they save money and are tasty too.

Tip
For accuracy when measuring the sorghum flour, use a 1-cup (250 mL) dry measure four times. Do not use a 4-cup (1 L) liquid measure, or you'll end up with extra sorghum flour in the mix.

NUTRITIONAL VALUE per serving

Calories	86
Fat, total	1 g
Fat, saturated	0 g
Cholesterol	0 mg
Sodium	204 mg
Carbohydrate	18 g
Fiber	2 g
Protein	2 g
Calcium	54 mg
Iron	2 mg

4 cups	sorghum flour	1 L
2⅔ cups	amaranth flour	650 mL
2 cups	whole bean flour	500 mL
1 cup	quinoa flour	250 mL
½ cup	ground flaxseed	125 mL
1 cup	potato starch	250 mL
½ cup	tapioca starch	125 mL
1½ cups	granulated sugar	375 mL
1 tbsp	xanthan gum	15 mL
¼ cup	GF baking powder	50 mL
2 tbsp	baking soda	25 mL
1 tbsp	salt	15 mL
3 tbsp	ground cinnamon	45 mL
½ tsp	ground allspice	2 mL
½ tsp	ground cloves	2 mL
½ tsp	ground ginger	2 mL

1. In a very large bowl, combine sorghum flour, amaranth flour, whole bean flour, quinoa flour, ground flaxseed, potato starch, tapioca starch, sugar, xanthan gum, baking powder, baking soda, salt, cinnamon, allspice, cloves and ginger. Mix well.

2. Immediately divide into 12 equal portions of approximately 1¼ cups (300 mL) each. Seal tightly in plastic bags, removing as much air as possible. Store at room temperature for up to 3 days or freeze for up to 6 months.

Variation
Substitute any type of bean or pea flour for the whole bean flour.

Small-Batch Make-Your-Own Muffin Mix

Makes about 3¾ cups (925 mL), or enough for 3 batches of 6 muffins each (1 muffin per serving)

We've received many requests for a small-batch muffin mix recipe from folks who enjoyed the recipes in our other gluten-free cookbooks, but who like lots of variety and/or live alone.

Tip
See page 164 for muffin mix tips.

1¼ cups	sorghum flour	300 mL
⅔ cup	amaranth flour	150 mL
½ cup	whole bean flour	125 mL
¼ cup	quinoa flour	50 mL
2 tbsp	ground flaxseed	25 mL
¼ cup	potato starch	50 mL
2 tbsp	tapioca starch	25 mL
⅓ cup	granulated sugar	75 mL
¾ tsp	xanthan gum	4 mL
1 tbsp	GF baking powder	15 mL
1½ tsp	baking soda	7 mL
¾ tsp	salt	4 mL
2¼ tsp	ground cinnamon	11 mL
⅛ tsp	ground allspice	0.5 mL
⅛ tsp	ground cloves	0.5 mL
⅛ tsp	ground ginger	0.5 mL

1. In a large bowl, combine sorghum flour, amaranth flour, whole bean flour, quinoa flour, ground flaxseed, potato starch, tapioca starch, sugar, xanthan gum, baking powder, baking soda, salt, cinnamon, allspice, cloves and ginger. Mix well.
2. Immediately divide into 3 equal portions of approximately 1¼ cups (300 mL) each. Seal tightly in plastic bags, removing as much air as possible. Store at room temperature for up to 3 days or freeze for up to 6 months.

Variation
Substitute any type of bean or pea flour for the whole bean flour.

NUTRITIONAL VALUE per serving
Calories	84
Fat, total	1 g
Fat, saturated	0 g
Cholesterol	0 mg
Sodium	204 mg
Carbohydrate	18 g
Fiber	2 g
Protein	2 g
Calcium	54 mg
Iron	2 mg

Banana Flaxseed Muffins

Makes 6 muffins (1 per serving)

Bananas and flaxseed form a great partnership in these muffins, with each flavor complementing the other.

Tips

The finer the flaxseed is cracked, the stronger the flaxseed flavor. We crack just slightly in a coffee mill. If you like a strong flax flavor, you'll really enjoy the egg-free version.

Purchase overripe bananas when you see them in the grocery store. Mash and freeze so they are ready when you need them. Thaw and bring to room temperature before using.

♦ 6-cup muffin tin, lightly greased

1	egg	1
1 cup	mashed banana	250 mL
2 tbsp	vegetable oil	25 mL
1 tbsp	freshly squeezed lemon juice	15 mL
1¼ cups	Make-Your-Own-Muffin Mix (see recipe, page 165) or Small-Batch Make-Your-Own Muffin Mix (see recipe, page 166)	300 mL
⅓ cup	flaxseed, cracked	75 mL

1. In a large bowl, using an electric mixer, beat egg, banana, oil and lemon juice until combined. Add muffin mix and flaxseed; mix just until combined.

2. Spoon batter evenly into each cup of prepared muffin tin. Let stand for 30 minutes. Meanwhile, preheat oven to 350°F (180°C). Bake for 18 to 20 minutes, or until firm to the touch. Remove from pan immediately and let cool completely on a rack.

To make this recipe egg-free

Omit egg from recipe. Combine 2 tbsp (25 mL) flax flour, ground flaxseed or ground Salba with 3 tbsp (45 mL) warm water. Let stand for 5 minutes. Add with liquid ingredients. Increase baking time by 2 to 3 minutes.

Variation

Raisins or nuts can be substituted for the cracked flaxseed.

NUTRITIONAL VALUE per serving	
Calories	210
Fat, total	10 g
Fat, saturated	1 g
Cholesterol	31 mg
Sodium	216 mg
Carbohydrate	29 g
Fiber	5 g
Protein	5 g
Calcium	80 mg
Iron	3 mg

Cranberry Applesauce Muffins

Makes 6 muffins (1 per serving)

These colorful muffins are an easy way to enjoy the flavor of applesauce with the contrasting tartness of cranberries.

Tip

To partially defrost the frozen cranberries, place in a single layer on a microwave-safe plate and microwave on High for 80 seconds.

♦ *6-cup muffin tin, lightly greased*

1	egg	1
¾ cup	unsweetened applesauce	175 mL
2 tbsp	vegetable oil	25 mL
1 tbsp	freshly squeezed lemon juice	15 mL
1¼ cups	Make-Your-Own-Muffin Mix (see recipe, page 165) or Small-Batch Make-Your-Own Muffin Mix (see recipe, page 166)	300 mL
1 cup	fresh or partially thawed frozen cranberries	250 mL

1. In a large bowl, using an electric mixer, beat egg, applesauce, oil and lemon juice until combined. Add muffin mix and mix just until combined. Stir in cranberries.

2. Spoon batter evenly into each cup of prepared muffin tin. Let stand for 30 minutes. Meanwhile, preheat oven to 350°F (180°C). Bake for 18 to 20 minutes, or until firm to the touch. Remove from pan immediately and let cool completely on a rack.

To make this recipe egg-free
Omit egg from recipe. Combine 2 tbsp (25 mL) flax flour, ground flaxseed or ground Salba with 2 tbsp (25 mL) warm water. Let stand for 5 minutes. Add with liquid ingredients. Increase baking time by 2 to 3 minutes.

Variation
Substitute coarsely chopped dried cherries for the cranberries.

NUTRITIONAL VALUE per serving	
Calories	158
Fat, total	6 g
Fat, saturated	1 g
Cholesterol	31 mg
Sodium	214 mg
Carbohydrate	24 g
Fiber	3 g
Protein	3 g
Calcium	60 mg
Iron	2 mg

Pineapple Nut Muffins

Makes 6 muffins (1 per serving)

The natural sweetness of the pineapple, along with its moist texture, makes these muffins an excellent addition to any lunch box.

Tip

Be sure to include plenty of juice when spooning the crushed pineapple into the measure.

♦ 6-cup muffin tin, lightly greased

1	egg	1
1 cup	crushed pineapple, including juice	250 mL
2 tbsp	vegetable oil	25 mL
1 tbsp	freshly squeezed lemon juice	15 mL
1 1/4 cups	Make-Your-Own-Muffin Mix (see recipe, page 165) or Small-Batch Make-Your-Own Muffin Mix (see recipe, page 166)	300 mL
1/2 cup	chopped walnuts	125 mL

1. In a large bowl, using an electric mixer, beat egg, pineapple, oil and lemon juice until combined. Add muffin mix and walnuts; mix just until combined.

2. Spoon batter evenly into each cup of prepared muffin tin. Let stand for 30 minutes. Meanwhile, preheat oven to 350°F (180°C). Bake for 18 to 20 minutes, or until firm to the touch. Remove from pan immediately and let cool completely on a rack.

To make this recipe egg-free
Omit egg from recipe. Combine 2 tbsp (25 mL) flax flour, ground flaxseed or ground Salba with 1/4 cup (50 mL) warm water. Let stand for 5 minutes. Add with liquid ingredients. Increase baking time by 2 to 3 minutes.

Variation

Substitute 1/4 cup (50 mL) shredded unsweetened coconut for half of the walnuts.

NUTRITIONAL VALUE per serving

Calories	225
Fat, total	13 g
Fat, saturated	1 g
Cholesterol	31 mg
Sodium	217 mg
Carbohydrate	25 g
Fiber	3 g
Protein	5 g
Calcium	68 mg
Iron	2 mg

Pumpkin Seed Muffins

**Makes 6 muffins
(1 per serving)**

Looking for a change
from traditional pumpkin
pie at Thanksgiving? Try
these muffins.

Tip

For information on
toasting seeds and nuts,
see the Technique
Glossary, page 301.

♦ *6-cup muffin tin, lightly greased*

1	egg	1
⅔ cup	canned pumpkin purée (not pie filling)	150 mL
2 tbsp	vegetable oil	25 mL
¼ cup	freshly squeezed orange juice	50 mL
1¼ cups	Make-Your-Own-Muffin Mix (see recipe, page 165) or Small-Batch Make-Your-Own Muffin Mix (see recipe, page 166)	300 mL
½ cup	green pumpkin seeds, toasted	125 mL
¼ cup	chopped pecans, toasted	50 mL

1. In a large bowl, using an electric mixer, beat egg, pumpkin, oil and orange juice until combined. Add muffin mix, pumpkin seeds and pecans; mix just until combined.

2. Spoon batter evenly into each cup of prepared muffin tin. Let stand for 30 minutes. Meanwhile, preheat oven to 350°F (180°C). Bake for 18 to 20 minutes, or until firm to the touch. Remove from pan immediately and let cool completely on a rack.

> **To make this recipe egg-free**
> Omit egg from recipe. Combine 2 tbsp (25 mL) flax flour, ground flaxseed or ground Salba with ¼ cup (50 mL) warm water. Let stand for 5 minutes. Add with liquid ingredients. Increase baking time by 2 to 3 minutes.

Variation

For a spicier muffin, add traditional pumpkin pie spices: ¼ tsp (1 mL) each ground ginger, nutmeg and cloves.

**NUTRITIONAL VALUE
per serving**

Calories	201
Fat, total	10 g
Fat, saturated	1 g
Cholesterol	31 mg
Sodium	216 mg
Carbohydrate	24 g
Fiber	3 g
Protein	5 g
Calcium	71 mg
Iron	3 mg

Breads and Spreads

continued on next page

Using Your Bread Machine

When it comes to baking, Murphy's Law is accurate: Anything that can go wrong will go wrong. Don't wait for your bread machine to bake an unacceptable loaf. Read the bread machine manual to become familiar with your make and model. Happy baking depends on it.

There is a great deal of variation among bread machines on the market today. Some models have a more vigorous and longer knead than others, resulting in slightly different loaves from the same recipe.

The recipes in this chapter are developed for either 1.5-lb (750 g) or 2-lb (1 kg) bread machines. The 2- to 3-lb (1 to 1.5 kg) bread machines with two kneading blades are too large to properly knead the amount of dough in the recipes.

When purchasing a new bread machine, make sure it has at least one of the following: a Rapid Cycle of 2 hours; both a Dough Cycle and a Bake Cycle; programmable cycles; or a dedicated Gluten-Free Cycle. Neither the 58-minute nor the 70-minute Rapid Cycle is long enough to rise and bake loaves successfully. If your bread machine doesn't have one of these four selections, try baking the loaves using a Basic, White or Sweet Cycle.

To Use the 2-Hour Rapid Cycle
Select the 2-Hour Rapid Cycle. Remove the kneading blade at the end of the long knead, then allow the cycle to finish.

To Use the Dough Cycle, then the Bake Cycle
Select the Dough Cycle. Remove the kneading blade at the end of the long knead, then allow the cycle to finish. Immediately select the Bake Cycle, setting it to 350°F or 360°F (180°C or 185°C) for 60 minutes. Allow the Bake Cycle to finish. (It is important to get to know your bread machine. We have one that is a lot hotter than the rest, and we have to lower the baking temperature to get a good result. In most machines, the default temperature is 350°F (180°C). Check your bread machine manual to learn how to change time and temperature.)

To Use Programmable Cycles
Set a short knead of 2 minutes (the machine stirs slowly, allowing for the addition of dry ingredients.) Then set a knead of 20 minutes, a rise of 70 minutes and a 60-minute Bake Cycle at 350°F (180°C). When prompted, set all other cycles to 0.

To Use the Dedicated Gluten-Free Cycle
Select the Gluten-Free Cycle. Remove the kneading blade when the machine signals or at the end of the long knead.

Tips for Bread Machine Baking

- If your bread machine has a Preheat Cycle, keep the top down until mixing starts so heat does not escape. As soon as the liquids begin to mix, add the dry ingredients, scraping the corners, sides and bottom of the baking pan and the kneading blade while adding. Watch that your rubber spatula does not get caught under the rotating blade. Continue scraping until no dry ingredients remain and dough is well mixed. Some machines require more "help" mixing than others.

- The consistency of the dough will be closer to that of a cake batter than a traditional yeast dough. You should see the motion of the kneading blade turning. The mixing mark of the kneading blade remains on top of the dough. Some doughs are thicker than others, but do not adjust by adding more liquid or dry ingredients.

- The kneading blade needs to be removed at the end of the long knead to prevent the collapse of the final loaf. Some bread machines knead intermittently rather than continuously, so the first few times you use a new machine, listen carefully for the sounds of the different cycles. Make notes of the times the cycles change. Then set an auxiliary timer for the time the kneading finishes and the rising starts. This will alert you to when to remove the kneading blade. The dough is sticky, so rinse the rubber spatula and your hand with cold water before removing the blade. Smooth the top of the loaf quickly.

- When we developed recipes for our first two GF cookbooks, we found we needed close to 1 tbsp (15 mL) of yeast for a quality loaf; however, using the new bread machine models on the market today, many of our original loaves now rise and collapse slightly during baking and cooling. If this happens when you're preparing a recipe from one of our earlier cookbooks, decrease the yeast by almost half the next time you prepare the recipe.

- Some bread machines and some recipes bake darker-colored crusts than others. If you find certain loaves too dark, next time set the Bake Cycle temperature lower. When baking on a Gluten-Free Cycle, a Basic Cycle or a 2-Hour Rapid Cycle, select a lighter crust setting.

- At the end of the baking cycle, before turning the machine off, take the temperature of the loaf using an instant-read thermometer. It should read 200°F (100°C). If it has not reached the recommended temperature, leave the loaf in the machine for 15 to 20 minutes on the Keep Warm Cycle.

- Slice the cooled loaf with an electric knife or bread knife with a serrated blade. Place one or two slices in individual plastic bags, then place bags in a larger resealable bag. Freeze for up to 3 weeks. Remove a slice or two at a time.

Tips for Mixer-Method Baking

- Select a heavy-duty mixer with a paddle attachment for the best mixing of ingredients.
- With the mixer set to medium speed, beat the dough for 4 minutes. Set a kitchen timer. You will be surprised how long 4 minutes seems when you are waiting.
- Fill the lightly greased pan only two-thirds full, then set, uncovered, in a warm draft-free place until the dough reaches the top of the pan. This usually takes 60 to 75 minutes. Be patient: the loaf rises a lot in the last 15 minutes of the rising time. Do not let the loaf over-rise, or it could collapse during baking.
- After baking, take the temperature of the loaf using an instant-read thermometer. It should read 200°F (100°C). If it doesn't, continue baking until it does, even if loaf is golden brown and looks baked. Remove loaf from pan and immediately place on a cooling rack to prevent a soggy loaf.

Make-Your-Own Bread Mixes

Sometimes you are just too busy to take the time to bake a loaf of bread. Just the thought of taking out and measuring the flour, sugar, seeds and grains seems like too much work. Wouldn't a mix be handy at these times?

You can make your own mixes from any of the recipes in this chapter. Here are some hints:

- Next time you bake a loaf, measure 3 or 4 extra sets of ingredients into plastic bags. Mixes should contain all the dry ingredients except the yeast; the extra exposure to air stales the yeast too quickly.
- Substitute granulated sugar for honey and brown sugar for molasses.
- Label your plastic bags with the recipe name and cycle to use, as well as the date. List on the label the amounts of ingredients that must be added to the mix to finish the loaf.
- The mix can be stored at room temperature for up to 3 weeks or frozen for up to 6 weeks. Bring to room temperature before using.
- Be sure to mix well to distribute the ingredients evenly before adding to baking pan.
- A bread machine mix with instructions for finishing, presented in a fancy wicker basket along with some jam and jelly, makes an excellent hostess gift.

Ancient Grains Bread
(Mixer Method)

Makes 15 slices (1 per serving)

Here's a quartet of healthy grains — sorghum, amaranth, cornmeal and quinoa — combined in a soft-textured, nutritious loaf that's perfect for sandwiches.

Tip

To ensure success, see page 175 for extra information on baking yeast bread using the mixer method.

♦ *9- by 5-inch (2 L) loaf pan, lightly greased*

1 cup	sorghum flour	250 mL
⅔ cup	amaranth flour	150 mL
½ cup	cornmeal	125 mL
¼ cup	quinoa flour	50 mL
⅓ cup	tapioca starch	75 mL
⅓ cup	packed brown sugar	75 mL
1 tbsp	xanthan gum	15 mL
1 tbsp	bread machine or instant yeast	15 mL
1½ tsp	salt	7 mL
2	eggs	2
1	egg white	1
1 cup	water	250 mL
2 tbsp	vegetable oil	25 mL
1 tsp	cider vinegar	5 mL

1. In a large bowl or plastic bag, combine sorghum flour, amaranth flour, cornmeal, quinoa flour, tapioca starch, brown sugar, xanthan gum, yeast and salt. Mix well and set aside.

2. In a separate bowl, using a heavy-duty electric mixer with paddle attachment, combine eggs, egg white, water, oil and vinegar until well blended. With the mixer on its lowest speed, slowly add the dry ingredients until combined. Stop the machine and scrape the bottom and sides of the bowl with a rubber spatula. With the mixer on medium speed, beat for 4 minutes.

3. Spoon into prepared pan. Let rise, uncovered, in a warm, draft-free place for 60 to 75 minutes, or until dough has risen to the top of the pan. Meanwhile, preheat oven to 350°F (180°C).

NUTRITIONAL VALUE
per serving

Calories	135
Fat, total	3 g
Fat, saturated	0 g
Cholesterol	25 mg
Sodium	248 mg
Carbohydrate	23 g
Fiber	2 g
Protein	4 g
Calcium	20 mg
Iron	2 mg

4. Bake for 35 to 45 minutes, or until loaf sounds hollow when tapped on the bottom. Remove from the pan immediately and let cool completely on a rack.

> **To make this recipe egg-free**
> Omit eggs and egg white from the recipe. Combine ⅓ cup (75 mL) flax flour or ground flaxseed with an additional ½ cup (125 mL) warm water. Set aside for 5 minutes. Add with the liquids. You may need to increase the baking time by 5 to 10 minutes.

Ancient Grains Bread
(Bread Machine Method)

Makes 15 slices (1 per serving)

Here's a quartet of healthy grains — sorghum, amaranth, cornmeal and quinoa — combined in a soft-textured, nutritious loaf that's perfect for sandwiches.

Tip

To ensure success, see page 174 for extra information on baking yeast bread in a bread machine.

1 cup	sorghum flour	250 mL
¾ cup	amaranth flour	175 mL
¾ cup	cornmeal	175 mL
¼ cup	quinoa flour	50 mL
½ cup	tapioca starch	125 mL
⅓ cup	packed brown sugar	75 mL
1 tbsp	xanthan gum	15 mL
¾ tsp	bread machine or instant yeast	4 mL
1½ tsp	salt	7 mL
1¼ cups	water	300 mL
2 tbsp	vegetable oil	25 mL
1 tsp	cider vinegar	5 mL
2	eggs, lightly beaten	2
2	egg whites, lightly beaten	2

1. In a large bowl or plastic bag, combine sorghum flour, amaranth flour, cornmeal, quinoa flour, tapioca starch, brown sugar, xanthan gum, yeast and salt. Mix well and set aside.

2. Pour water, oil and vinegar into the bread machine baking pan. Add eggs and egg whites.

3. Select the **Dough Cycle**. As the bread machine is mixing, gradually add the dry ingredients, scraping bottom and sides of pan with a rubber spatula. Try to incorporate all the dry ingredients within 1 to 2 minutes. When the mixing and kneading are complete, remove the kneading blade, leaving the bread pan in the bread machine. Quickly smooth the top of the loaf. Allow the cycle to finish. Turn off the bread machine.

NUTRITIONAL VALUE per serving	
Calories	151
Fat, total	3 g
Fat, saturated	0 g
Cholesterol	25 mg
Sodium	252 mg
Carbohydrate	27 g
Fiber	2 g
Protein	4 g
Calcium	21 mg
Iron	2 mg

Tip

Substitute $1/4$ cup (50 mL) liquid egg whites for the egg whites and $1/2$ cup (125 mL) liquid eggs for the whole eggs.

4. Select the **Bake Cycle**. Set time to 60 minutes and temperature to 350°F (180°C). Allow the cycle to finish. Remove loaf from the pan immediately and let cool completely on a rack.

> **To make this recipe egg-free**
> Omit eggs and egg whites from the recipe. Add 4 tsp (20 mL) powdered egg replacer with the dry ingredients. Increase yeast to 2 tsp (10 mL). Increase water by $1/4$ cup (50 mL). This flavorful egg-free loaf is shorter than some.

Applesauce Apple Oatmeal Bread (Mixer Method)

This sweetly spiced loaf is flavored with apple cider and applesauce. Serve it spread with Apple Butter (page 232).

Tip

To ensure success, see page 175 for extra information on baking yeast bread using the mixer method.

NUTRITIONAL VALUE per serving	
Calories	112
Fat, total	3 g
Fat, saturated	0 g
Cholesterol	13 mg
Sodium	204 mg
Carbohydrate	19 g
Fiber	2 g
Protein	3 g
Calcium	12 mg
Iron	1 mg

◆ *9- by 5-inch (2 L) loaf pan, lightly greased*

1½ cups	sorghum flour	375 mL
½ cup	GF oats	125 mL
⅓ cup	GF oat flour	75 mL
⅓ cup	tapioca starch	75 mL
2 tbsp	packed brown sugar	25 mL
2½ tsp	xanthan gum	12 mL
2 tsp	bread machine or instant yeast	10 mL
1¼ tsp	salt	6 mL
1 tsp	apple pie spice	5 mL
1	egg	1
1	egg white	1
⅔ cup	apple cider	150 mL
½ cup	unsweetened applesauce	125 mL
2 tbsp	vegetable oil	25 mL

1. In a large bowl or plastic bag, combine sorghum flour, oats, oat flour, tapioca starch, brown sugar, xanthan gum, yeast, salt and apple pie spice. Mix well and set aside.

2. In a separate bowl, using a heavy-duty electric mixer with paddle attachment, combine egg, egg white, apple cider, applesauce and oil until well blended. With the mixer on its lowest speed, slowly add the dry ingredients until combined. Stop the machine and scrape the bottom and sides of the bowl with a rubber spatula. With the mixer on medium speed, beat for 4 minutes.

3. Spoon into prepared pan. Let rise, uncovered, in a warm, draft-free place for 60 to 75 minutes, or until dough has risen almost to the top of the pan. Meanwhile, preheat oven to 350°F (180°C).

If the apple cider and applesauce are cold from the refrigerator, allow an additional 15 minutes of rising time, or warm them to room temperature before adding.

4. Bake for 35 to 45 minutes, or until loaf sounds hollow when tapped on the bottom. Remove from the pan immediately and let cool completely on a rack.

To make this recipe egg-free

Omit egg and egg white from recipe. Combine $1/3$ cup (75 mL) flax flour or ground flaxseed with an additional $1/3$ cup (75 mL) warm apple cider. Set aside for 5 minutes. Add with the liquids. You may need to increase the baking time by 5 to 10 minutes.

Variations

Substitute $1/2$ tsp (2 mL) ground cinnamon, $1/4$ tsp (1 mL) ground nutmeg and a pinch each of ground allspice and ground cloves or ground ginger for the apple pie spice.

For a tasty sandwich bread, omit the apple pie spice.

Applesauce Apple Oatmeal Bread (Bread Machine Method)

Makes 15 slices (1 per serving)

This sweetly spiced loaf is flavored with apple cider and applesauce. Serve it spread with Apple Butter (page 232).

Tip

To ensure success, see page 174 for extra information on baking yeast bread in a bread machine.

1⅓ cups	sorghum flour	325 mL
½ cup	GF oats	125 mL
½ cup	GF oat flour	125 mL
⅓ cup	tapioca starch	75 mL
3 tbsp	packed brown sugar	45 mL
1 tbsp	xanthan gum	15 mL
1 tbsp	bread machine or instant yeast	15 mL
1½ tsp	salt	7 mL
1½ tsp	apple pie spice	7 mL
¾ cup	apple cider	175 mL
½ cup	unsweetened applesauce	125 mL
2 tbsp	vegetable oil	25 mL
2	eggs, lightly beaten	2

1. In a large bowl or plastic bag, combine sorghum flour, oats, oat flour, tapioca starch, brown sugar, xanthan gum, yeast, salt and apple pie spice. Mix well and set aside.

2. Pour apple cider, applesauce and oil into the bread machine baking pan. Add eggs.

3. Select the **Dough Cycle**. As the bread machine is mixing, gradually add the dry ingredients, scraping bottom and sides of pan with a rubber spatula. Try to incorporate all the dry ingredients within 1 to 2 minutes. When the mixing and kneading are complete, remove the kneading blade, leaving the bread pan in the bread machine. Quickly smooth the top of the loaf. Allow the cycle to finish. Turn off the bread machine.

NUTRITIONAL VALUE per serving	
Calories	133
Fat, total	3 g
Fat, saturated	0 g
Cholesterol	25 mg
Sodium	244 mg
Carbohydrate	23 g
Fiber	2 g
Protein	4 g
Calcium	16 mg
Iron	2 mg

Tip

If the apple cider and applesauce are cold from the refrigerator, allow an additional 15 minutes of rising time, or warm them to room temperature before adding.

4. Select the **Bake Cycle**. Set time to 60 minutes and temperature to 350°F (180°C). Allow the cycle to finish. Remove loaf from the pan immediately and let cool completely on a rack.

> **To make this recipe egg-free**
> Omit eggs from the recipe. Combine $\frac{1}{3}$ cup (75 mL) flax flour or ground flaxseed with an additional $\frac{1}{2}$ cup (125 mL) warm apple cider. Set aside for 5 minutes. Add with the liquids.

Variations

Substitute $\frac{3}{4}$ tsp (4 mL) ground cinnamon, $\frac{1}{2}$ tsp (2 mL) ground nutmeg and a pinch each of ground allspice and ground cloves or ground ginger for the apple pie spice.

For a tasty sandwich bread, omit the apple pie spice.

Fruited Mock Pumpernickel Loaf (Mixer Method)

This moist, rich, dark bread is a favorite of our 93-year-old German-born neighbor. With the sweetness of apricots and dates, it's perfect with fresh fruit for lunch.

Tips

To ensure success, see page 175 for extra information on baking yeast bread using the mixer method.

Snip dates and apricots with kitchen shears. Dip shears in warm water when they become sticky.

NUTRITIONAL VALUE per serving	
Calories	147
Fat, total	4 g
Fat, saturated	0 g
Cholesterol	25 mg
Sodium	244 mg
Carbohydrate	26 g
Fiber	2 g
Protein	3 g
Calcium	21 mg
Iron	1 mg

♦ *9- by 5-inch (2 L) loaf pan, lightly greased*

1 cup	sorghum flour	250 mL
½ cup	pea flour	125 mL
⅓ cup	cornstarch	75 mL
¼ cup	tapioca starch	50 mL
2 tbsp	packed brown sugar	25 mL
1 tbsp	xanthan gum	15 mL
2 tsp	bread machine or instant yeast	10 mL
1½ tsp	salt	7 mL
2 tsp	instant coffee granules	10 mL
2 tsp	unsweetened cocoa powder, sifted	10 mL
2	eggs	2
1¼ cups	water	300 mL
3 tbsp	vegetable oil	45 mL
2 tbsp	fancy molasses	25 mL
1 tsp	cider vinegar	5 mL
½ cup	snipped dried apricots	125 mL
½ cup	coarsely chopped pitted dates	125 mL

1. In a large bowl or plastic bag, combine sorghum flour, pea flour, cornstarch, tapioca starch, brown sugar, xanthan gum, yeast, salt, coffee granules and cocoa. Mix well and set aside.

2. In a separate bowl, using a heavy-duty electric mixer with paddle attachment, combine eggs, water, oil, molasses and vinegar until well blended. With the mixer on its lowest speed, slowly add the dry ingredients until combined. Stop the machine and scrape the bottom and sides of the bowl with a rubber spatula. With the mixer on medium speed, beat for 4 minutes. Stir in apricots and dates.

Tips

Pea flour, like soy flour, has a distinctive odor when wet that disappears with baking.

Tent with foil partway through the baking time, as this is a very dark-colored loaf.

3. Spoon into prepared pan. Let rise, uncovered, in a warm, draft-free place for 60 to 75 minutes, or until dough has risen to the top of the pan. Meanwhile, preheat oven to 350°F (180°C) with rack set in bottom third of oven.

4. Bake for 35 to 45 minutes, tenting with foil partway through, or until loaf sounds hollow when tapped on the bottom. Remove from the pan immediately and let cool completely on a rack.

To make this recipe egg-free
Omit eggs from the recipe. Combine $\frac{1}{3}$ cup (75 mL) flax flour or ground flaxseed with an additional $\frac{1}{3}$ cup (75 mL) warm water. Set aside for 5 minutes. Add with the liquids. You may need to increase the baking time by 5 to 10 minutes.

Variations
Substitute chopped prunes or figs for the dates and dried apples for the apricots.

Any type of bean flour can be substituted for the pea flour.

Fruited Mock Pumpernickel Loaf (Bread Machine Method)

Makes 15 slices (1 per serving)

This moist, rich, dark bread is a favorite of our 93-year-old German-born neighbor. With the sweetness of apricots and dates, it's perfect with fresh fruit for lunch.

Tips

To ensure success, see page 174 for extra information on baking yeast bread in a bread machine.

Snip dates and apricots with kitchen shears. Dip shears in warm water when they become sticky.

1¼ cups	sorghum flour	300 mL
1 cup	pea flour	250 mL
½ cup	cornstarch	125 mL
⅓ cup	tapioca starch	75 mL
3 tbsp	packed brown sugar	45 mL
1 tbsp	xanthan gum	15 mL
1 tsp	bread machine or instant yeast	5 mL
1½ tsp	salt	7 mL
2 tsp	instant coffee granules	10 mL
2 tsp	unsweetened cocoa powder, sifted	10 mL
½ cup	snipped dried apricots	125 mL
½ cup	coarsely chopped pitted dates	125 mL
1⅔ cups	water	400 mL
2 tbsp	vegetable oil	25 mL
3 tbsp	fancy molasses	45 mL
1 tsp	cider vinegar	5 mL
3	eggs, lightly beaten	3

1. In a large bowl or plastic bag, combine sorghum flour, pea flour, cornstarch, tapioca starch, brown sugar, xanthan gum, yeast, salt, coffee granules, cocoa, apricots and dates. Mix well and set aside.

2. Pour water, oil, molasses and vinegar into the bread machine baking pan. Add eggs.

3. Select the **Dough Cycle**. As the bread machine is mixing, gradually add the dry ingredients, scraping bottom and sides of pan with a rubber spatula. Try to incorporate all the dry ingredients within 1 to 2 minutes. When the mixing and kneading are complete, remove the kneading blade, leaving the bread pan in the bread machine. Quickly smooth the top of the loaf. Allow the cycle to finish. Turn off the bread machine.

NUTRITIONAL VALUE per serving	
Calories	180
Fat, total	3 g
Fat, saturated	0 g
Cholesterol	37 mg
Sodium	250 mg
Carbohydrate	34 g
Fiber	3 g
Protein	5 g
Calcium	29 mg
Iron	2 mg

Tip

Pea flour, like soy flour, has a distinctive odor when wet that disappears with baking.

4. Select the **Bake Cycle**. Set time to 60 minutes and temperature to 350°F (180°C). Allow the cycle to finish. Remove loaf from the pan immediately and let cool completely on a rack.

To make this recipe egg-free
Omit eggs from the recipe. Combine $\frac{1}{2}$ cup (125 mL) flax flour or ground flaxseed with an additional $\frac{1}{2}$ cup (125 mL) warm water. Set aside for 5 minutes. Add with the liquids.

Variations

Substitute chopped prunes or figs for the dates and dried apples for the apricots.

Any type of bean flour can be substituted for the pea flour.

Honeyed Walnut Bread
(Mixer Method)

**Makes 15 slices
(1 per serving)**

Enhance the nutty walnut flavor of this basic brown sandwich or breakfast bread by toasting individual slices.

Tips

To ensure success, see page 175 for extra information on baking yeast bread using the mixer method.

Store brown rice flour and rice bran in the refrigerator.

♦ 9- by 5-inch (2 L) loaf pan, lightly greased

1¼ cups	sorghum flour	300 mL
½ cup	brown rice flour	125 mL
⅓ cup	cornstarch	75 mL
⅓ cup	rice bran	75 mL
1 tbsp	xanthan gum	15 mL
1 tbsp	bread machine or instant yeast	15 mL
1½ tsp	salt	7 mL
¾ cup	coarsely chopped walnuts, toasted (see tip, opposite)	175 mL
2	eggs	2
1	egg white	1
1 cup	water	250 mL
3 tbsp	walnut oil	45 mL
⅓ cup	liquid honey	75 mL
1 tsp	cider vinegar	5 mL

1. In a large bowl or plastic bag, combine sorghum flour, brown rice flour, cornstarch, rice bran, xanthan gum, yeast, salt and walnuts. Mix well and set aside.

2. In a separate bowl, using a heavy-duty electric mixer with paddle attachment, combine eggs, egg white, water, walnut oil, honey and vinegar until well blended. With the mixer on its lowest speed, slowly add the dry ingredients until combined. Stop the machine and scrape the bottom and sides of the bowl with a rubber spatula. With the mixer on medium speed, beat for 4 minutes.

3. Spoon into prepared pan. Let rise, uncovered, in a warm, draft-free place for 60 to 75 minutes, or until dough has risen to the top of the pan. Meanwhile, preheat oven to 350°F (180°C).

4. Bake for 35 to 45 minutes, or until loaf sounds hollow when tapped on the bottom. Remove from the pan immediately and let cool completely on a rack.

**NUTRITIONAL VALUE
per serving**

Calories	167
Fat, total	7 g
Fat, saturated	1 g
Cholesterol	25 mg
Sodium	246 mg
Carbohydrate	23 g
Fiber	2 g
Protein	4 g
Calcium	15 mg
Iron	2 mg

Tip

It's worth the time to toast the walnuts (for instructions, see under Nuts in the Technique Glossary, page 301). No need to let them cool; just add to the dry ingredients. Toast more walnuts than you need for this recipe. Cool and store the extra in a resealable plastic bag in the refrigerator.

To make this recipe egg-free

Omit eggs and egg white from the recipe. Combine ⅓ cup (75 mL) flax flour or ground flaxseed with an additional ½ cup (125 mL) warm water. Let stand for 5 minutes. Add with the liquids. You may need to increase the baking time by 5 to 10 minutes.

Variations

Substitute vegetable oil for the walnut oil.

If you cannot tolerate corn, substitute tapioca starch for the cornstarch.

Honeyed Walnut Bread
(Bread Machine Method)

Makes 15 slices (1 per serving)

Enhance the nutty walnut flavor of this basic brown sandwich or breakfast bread by toasting individual slices.

Tips

To ensure success, see page 174 for extra information on baking yeast bread in a bread machine.

Store brown rice flour and rice bran in the refrigerator.

Substitute ¼ cup (50 mL) liquid egg whites for the 2 egg whites and ½ cup (125 mL) liquid eggs for the whole eggs.

1½ cups	sorghum flour	375 mL
¾ cup	brown rice flour	175 mL
½ cup	cornstarch	125 mL
½ cup	rice bran	125 mL
1 tbsp	xanthan gum	15 mL
1½ tsp	bread machine or instant yeast	7 mL
1½ tsp	salt	7 mL
1 cup	coarsely chopped walnuts, toasted (see tip, at left)	250 mL
1¼ cups	water	300 mL
2 tbsp	walnut oil	25 mL
⅓ cup	liquid honey	75 mL
1 tsp	cider vinegar	5 mL
2	eggs, lightly beaten	2
2	egg whites, lightly beaten	2

1. In a large bowl or plastic bag, combine sorghum flour, brown rice flour, cornstarch, rice bran, xanthan gum, yeast, salt and walnuts. Mix well and set aside.

2. Pour water, walnut oil, honey and vinegar into the bread machine baking pan. Add eggs and egg whites.

3. Select the **Dough Cycle**. As the bread machine is mixing, gradually add the dry ingredients, scraping bottom and sides of pan with a rubber spatula. Try to incorporate all the dry ingredients within 1 to 2 minutes. When the mixing and kneading are complete, remove the kneading blade, leaving the bread pan in the bread machine. Quickly smooth the top of the loaf. Allow the cycle to finish. Turn off the bread machine.

4. Select the **Bake Cycle**. Set time to 60 minutes and temperature to 350°F (180°C). Allow the cycle to finish. Remove loaf from the pan immediately and let cool completely on a rack.

NUTRITIONAL VALUE per serving

Calories	215
Fat, total	9 g
Fat, saturated	1 g
Cholesterol	25 mg
Sodium	251 mg
Carbohydrate	30 g
Fiber	3 g
Protein	5 g
Calcium	18 mg
Iron	2 mg

Tip

It's worth the time to toast the walnuts (for instructions, see under Nuts in the Technique Glossary, page 301). No need to let them cool; just add to the dry ingredients. Toast more walnuts than you need for this recipe. Cool and store the extra in a resealable plastic bag in the refrigerator.

To make this recipe egg-free

Omit eggs and egg whites from recipe. Combine $1/3$ cup (75 mL) flax flour or ground flaxseed with an additional $1/2$ cup (125 mL) warm water. Set aside for 5 minutes. Add with the liquids.

Variations

Substitute vegetable oil for the walnut oil.

If you cannot tolerate corn, substitute tapioca starch for the cornstarch.

Roasted Garlic Potato Bread (Mixer Method)

Makes 15 slices (1 per serving)

This flavorful loaf with a warm, creamy color is a perfect accompaniment to soup on a cold winter's night.

Tips

To ensure success, see page 175 for extra information on baking yeast bread using the mixer method.

For information on roasting garlic, see the Technique Glossary, page 300.

◆ 9- by 5-inch (2 L) loaf pan, lightly greased

1 cup	brown rice flour	250 mL
¾ cup	almond flour	175 mL
½ cup	amaranth flour	125 mL
¼ cup	potato starch	50 mL
1 tbsp	xanthan gum	15 mL
1 tbsp	bread machine or instant yeast	15 mL
1½ tsp	salt	7 mL
⅓ cup	instant potato flakes	75 mL
2	eggs	2
1	egg white	1
1¼ cups	water	300 mL
2 tbsp	extra-virgin olive oil	25 mL
3	cloves roasted garlic	3
3 tbsp	liquid honey	45 mL
1 tsp	cider vinegar	5 mL

1. In a large bowl or plastic bag, combine brown rice flour, almond flour, amaranth flour, potato starch, xanthan gum, yeast, salt and potato flakes. Mix well and set aside.

2. In a separate bowl, using a heavy-duty electric mixer with paddle attachment, combine eggs, egg white, water, olive oil, garlic, honey and vinegar until well blended. With the mixer on its lowest speed, slowly add the dry ingredients until combined. Stop the machine and scrape the bottom and sides of the bowl with a rubber spatula. With the mixer on medium speed, beat for 4 minutes.

3. Spoon into prepared pan. Let rise, uncovered, in a warm, draft-free place for 60 to 75 minutes, or until dough has risen to the top of the pan. Meanwhile, preheat oven to 350°F (180°C).

NUTRITIONAL VALUE per serving	
Calories	139
Fat, total	6 g
Fat, saturated	1 g
Cholesterol	25 mg
Sodium	249 mg
Carbohydrate	19 g
Fiber	2 g
Protein	4 g
Calcium	27 mg
Iron	2 mg

Normally, garlic and yeast are enemies; however, they get along well after garlic is roasted. Still, even roasted garlic inhibits the action of the yeast, so avoid the temptation to use more than 3 cloves. Too much garlic, and the loaf will be short and heavy.

4. Bake for 35 to 45 minutes, or until loaf sounds hollow when tapped on the bottom. Remove from the pan immediately and let cool completely on a rack

---

To make this recipe egg-free

Omit eggs and egg white from the recipe. Add 4 tsp (20 mL) powdered egg replacer with the dry ingredients. Add an additional $\frac{1}{3}$ cup (75 mL) water. Spoon into 2 lightly greased $5\frac{1}{2}$- by 3-inch (500 mL) mini loaf pans and bake for 30 to 35 minutes.

Variations

Substitute $\frac{1}{3}$ cup (75 mL) mashed potato for the instant potato flakes. Add with the liquids.

For a stronger, more prominent garlic flavor, serve toasted or warmed with either a garlic butter or a garlic-flavored spread.

Potato Chive Bread: Omit the roasted garlic and add $\frac{1}{4}$ cup (50 mL) snipped fresh parsley and $\frac{1}{3}$ cup (75 mL) snipped fresh chives with the liquids.

Potato Dill Bread: Omit the roasted garlic and add $\frac{1}{4}$ cup (50 mL) snipped fresh dill with the liquids.

Roasted Garlic Potato Bread
(Bread Machine Method)

Makes 15 slices (1 per serving)

This flavorful loaf with a warm, creamy color is a perfect accompaniment to soup on a cold winter's night.

Tips

To ensure success, see page 174 for extra information on baking yeast bread in a bread machine.

For information on roasting garlic, see the Technique Glossary, page 300.

1 cup	brown rice flour	250 mL
1 cup	almond flour	250 mL
½ cup	amaranth flour	125 mL
⅓ cup	potato starch	75 mL
1 tbsp	xanthan gum	15 mL
1¾ tsp	bread machine or instant yeast	8 mL
1½ tsp	salt	7 mL
½ cup	instant potato flakes	125 mL
1⅓ cups	water	325 mL
2 tbsp	extra-virgin olive oil	25 mL
3 tbsp	liquid honey	45 mL
1 tsp	cider vinegar	5 mL
3	cloves roasted garlic (see tips, at left)	3
2	eggs, lightly beaten	2
2	egg whites, lightly beaten	2

1. In a large bowl or plastic bag, combine brown rice flour, almond flour, amaranth flour, potato starch, xanthan gum, yeast, salt and potato flakes. Mix well and set aside.

2. Pour water, olive oil, honey, vinegar and garlic into the bread machine baking pan. Add eggs and egg whites.

3. Select the **Dough Cycle**. As the bread machine is mixing, gradually add the dry ingredients, scraping bottom and sides of pan with a rubber spatula. Try to incorporate all the dry ingredients within 1 to 2 minutes. When the mixing and kneading are complete, remove the kneading blade, leaving the bread pan in the bread machine. Quickly smooth the top of the loaf. Allow the cycle to finish. Turn off the bread machine.

4. Select the **Bake Cycle**. Set time to 60 minutes and temperature to 350°F (180°C). Allow the cycle to finish. Remove loaf from the pan immediately and let cool completely on a rack.

NUTRITIONAL VALUE
per serving

Calories	154
Fat, total	7 g
Fat, saturated	1 g
Cholesterol	25 mg
Sodium	254 mg
Carbohydrate	20 g
Fiber	2 g
Protein	5 g
Calcium	32 mg
Iron	2 mg

Tip

Normally, garlic and yeast are enemies; however, they get along well after garlic is roasted. Still, even roasted garlic inhibits the action of the yeast, so avoid the temptation to use more than 3 cloves. Too much garlic, and the loaf will be short and heavy.

Variations

Substitute ⅓ cup (75 mL) mashed potato for the instant potato flakes. Add with the liquids.

For a stronger, more prominent garlic flavor, serve toasted or warmed with either a garlic butter or a garlic-flavored spread.

Potato Chive Bread: Omit the roasted garlic and add ¼ cup (50 mL) snipped fresh parsley and ⅓ cup (75 mL) snipped fresh chives with the liquids.

Potato Dill Bread: Omit the roasted garlic and add ¼ cup (50 mL) snipped fresh dill with the liquids.

Sunflower Flax Bread
(Mixer Method)

Looking for something different for your morning toast? Try this crunchy, nutty loaf with Pumpkin Spread (page 234).

Tips

To ensure success, see page 175 for extra information on baking yeast bread using the mixer method.

For information on cracking flaxseed, see the Technique Glossary, page 300.

NUTRITIONAL VALUE per serving	
Calories	155
Fat, total	10 g
Fat, saturated	1 g
Cholesterol	25 mg
Sodium	209 mg
Carbohydrate	19 g
Fiber	4 g
Protein	5 g
Calcium	40 mg
Iron	2 mg

♦ 9- by 5-inch (2 L) loaf pan, lightly greased

⅔ cup	sorghum flour	150 mL
½ cup	amaranth flour	125 mL
¼ cup	flax flour	50 mL
½ cup	potato starch	125 mL
¼ cup	cornstarch	50 mL
3 tbsp	granulated sugar	45 mL
2½ tsp	xanthan gum	12 mL
1 tbsp	bread machine or instant yeast	15 mL
1¼ tsp	salt	6 mL
½ cup	cracked flaxseed	125 mL
½ cup	raw unsalted sunflower seeds	125 mL
2	eggs	2
1	egg white	1
1 cup	water	250 mL
¼ cup	vegetable oil	50 mL
2 tsp	cider vinegar	10 mL

1. In a large bowl or plastic bag, combine sorghum flour, amaranth flour, flax flour, potato starch, cornstarch, sugar, xanthan gum, yeast, salt, flaxseed and sunflower seeds. Mix well and set aside.

2. In a separate bowl, using a heavy-duty electric mixer with paddle attachment, combine eggs, egg white, water, oil and vinegar until well blended. With the mixer on its lowest speed, slowly add the dry ingredients until combined. Stop the machine and scrape the bottom and sides of the bowl with a rubber spatula. With the mixer on medium speed, beat for 4 minutes.

3. Spoon into prepared pan. Let rise, uncovered, in a warm, draft-free place for 60 to 75 minutes, or until dough has risen to the top of the pan. Meanwhile, preheat oven to 350°F (180°C).

We tried this bread with sprouted flax powder, flax meal, ground flaxseed and flax flour. All yielded acceptable loaves.

4. Bake for 35 to 45 minutes, or until loaf sounds hollow when tapped on the bottom. Remove from the pan immediately and let cool completely on a rack.

To make this recipe egg-free
Omit eggs and egg white from the recipe. Combine $1/3$ cup (75 mL) flax flour or ground flaxseed with an additional $1/2$ cup (125 mL) warm water. Set aside for 5 minutes. Add with the liquids. You may need to increase the baking time by 5 to 10 minutes.

Variation
Substitute raw hemp powder for the flax flour and Hemp Hearts for the flaxseed.

Sunflower Flax Bread
(Bread Machine Method)

Looking for something different for your morning toast? Try this crunchy, nutty loaf with Pumpkin Spread (page 234).

Tips

To ensure success, see page 174 for extra information on baking yeast bread in a bread machine.

◆

For information on cracking flaxseed, see the Technique Glossary, page 300.

¾ cup	sorghum flour	175 mL
⅔ cup	amaranth flour	150 mL
⅓ cup	flax flour	75 mL
⅔ cup	potato starch	150 mL
⅓ cup	cornstarch	75 mL
¼ cup	granulated sugar	50 mL
2½ tsp	xanthan gum	12 mL
2 tsp	bread machine or instant yeast	10 mL
1½ tsp	salt	7 mL
½ cup	cracked flaxseed	125 mL
½ cup	raw unsalted sunflower seeds	125 mL
1¼ cups	water	300 mL
3 tbsp	vegetable oil	45 mL
2 tsp	cider vinegar	10 mL
2	eggs, lightly beaten	2
2	egg whites, lightly beaten	2

1. In a large bowl or plastic bag, combine sorghum flour, amaranth flour, flax flour, potato starch, cornstarch, sugar, xanthan gum, yeast, salt, flaxseed and sunflower seeds. Mix well and set aside.

2. Pour water, oil and vinegar into the bread machine baking pan. Add eggs and egg whites.

3. Select the **Dough Cycle**. As the bread machine is mixing, gradually add the dry ingredients, scraping bottom and sides of pan with a rubber spatula. Try to incorporate all the dry ingredients within 1 to 2 minutes. When the mixing and kneading are complete, remove the kneading blade, leaving the bread pan in the bread machine. Quickly smooth the top of the loaf. Allow the cycle to finish. Turn off the bread machine.

NUTRITIONAL VALUE per serving	
Calories	189
Fat, total	10 g
Fat, saturated	1 g
Cholesterol	25 mg
Sodium	252 mg
Carbohydrate	23 g
Fiber	4 g
Protein	11 g
Calcium	39 mg
Iron	3 mg

Tip

We tried this bread with sprouted flax powder, flax meal, ground flaxseed and flax flour. All yielded acceptable loaves.

4. Select the **Bake Cycle**. Set time to 60 minutes and temperature to 350°F (180°C). Allow the cycle to finish. Remove loaf from the pan immediately and let cool completely on a rack.

Variation

Substitute raw hemp powder for the flax flour and Hemp Hearts for the flaxseed.

Sourdough Starter

**Makes 3½ cups
(875 mL)
(1 cup/250 mL
per serving)**

You've been asking us for a sourdough bread with a tangy taste. Begin by making this starter, and you'll be on your way to enjoying gluten-free sourdough breads.

Tips

If the starter liquid turns green, pink or orange — or develops mold — throw it out and start again.

During hot weather, use a triple layer of cheesecloth to cover the sourdough starter when it is at room temperature. A loose-fitting lid on a large casserole dish works well too.

3 cups	warm water	750 mL
2 tbsp	granulated sugar	25 mL
2 tbsp	instant or bread machine yeast	25 mL
3 cups	sorghum flour	750 mL

1. In a very large glass bowl, combine water and sugar. Sprinkle with yeast, gently stir to moisten and let stand for 10 minutes.

2. Add sorghum flour and whisk until smooth.

3. Cover with a double layer of cheesecloth or a loose-fitting lid. Secure so that it is not touching the starter. Let stand at room temperature for 2 to 4 days, stirring 2 to 3 times a day. When ready to use, starter has a sour smell, with small bubbles rising to the surface.

4. Store, loosely covered, in the refrigerator until needed. If not used regularly, stir in 1 tsp (5 mL) granulated sugar every 10 days.

NUTRITIONAL VALUE per serving	
Calories	536
Fat, total	4 g
Fat, saturated	0 g
Cholesterol	0 mg
Sodium	9 mg
Carbohydrate	111 g
Fiber	14 g
Protein	19 g
Calcium	46 mg
Iron	7 mg

Tips for Successful Starters

Using the Starter

- It is normal for a starter to separate. The grayish liquid rises to the top, while the very thick part settles to the bottom of the storage container. Stir well before each use.
- The starter should have the consistency of pancake batter. If it's too thick, add a small amount of water before measuring. Bring the starter to room temperature by placing it in a bowl of hot water for 15 minutes before measuring.
- Until the starter becomes established and is working well, remove only 1 cup (250 mL) at a time.
- Make sure all utensils and pans that come into contact with the starter go through the dishwasher or are rinsed with a mild solution of water and bleach.

Feeding the Starter

- To replace each cup (250 mL) of starter used in preparing a recipe, add ¾ cup (175 mL) water, ¾ cup (175 mL) sorghum flour and 1 tsp (5 mL) granulated sugar to the remaining starter. Stir well, cover with a double layer of cheesecloth or a loose-fitting lid and let stand at room temperature for at least 24 hours, or until bubbly and sour smelling. Refrigerate, loosely covered.
- If not used regularly, stir in 1 tsp (5 mL) granulated sugar every 10 days.

Sourdough Loaf
(Mixer Method)

Try this warm creamy loaf the next time you feel like eating a sandwich.

Tip

To ensure success, see page 175 for extra information on baking yeast bread using the mixer method and read "Tips for Successful Starters," page 201.

◆ 9- by 5- inch (2 L) loaf pan, lightly greased

1 cup	brown rice flour	250 mL
¾ cup	amaranth flour	175 mL
⅓ cup	potato starch	75 mL
2 tbsp	granulated sugar	25 mL
1 tbsp	xanthan gum	15 mL
1 tbsp	bread machine or instant yeast	15 mL
1½ tsp	salt	7 mL
2	egg whites	2
1	egg	1
1 cup	Sourdough Starter (see recipe, page 200), at room temperature	250 mL
¼ cup	water	50 mL
2 tbsp	vegetable oil	25 mL

1. In a large bowl or plastic bag, combine brown rice flour, amaranth flour, potato starch, sugar, xanthan gum, yeast and salt. Mix well and set aside.

2. In a separate bowl, using a heavy-duty electric mixer with paddle attachment, combine egg whites, egg, sourdough starter, water and oil until well blended. With the mixer on its lowest speed, slowly add the dry ingredients until combined. Stop the machine and scrape the bottom and sides of the bowl with a rubber spatula. With the mixer on medium speed, beat for 4 minutes.

3. Spoon into prepared pan. Let rise, uncovered, in a warm, draft-free place for 60 to 80 minutes, or until dough has risen to the top of the pan. Meanwhile, preheat oven to 350°F (180°C).

4. Bake for 35 to 45 minutes, or until loaf sounds hollow when tapped on the bottom. Remove from the pan immediately and let cool completely on a rack.

NUTRITIONAL VALUE per serving	
Calories	139
Fat, total	3 g
Fat, saturated	0 g
Cholesterol	13 mg
Sodium	246 mg
Carbohydrate	24 g
Fiber	3 g
Protein	4 g
Calcium	15 mg
Iron	2 mg

Tip

Don't forget about the sourdough starter sitting in your refrigerator. If you haven't used it to make a loaf in the last 10 days, see page 201 for information on feeding it.

To make this recipe egg-free

Omit egg whites and egg from recipe. Combine $\frac{1}{2}$ cup (125 mL) flax flour or ground flaxseed with an additional $\frac{3}{4}$ cup (175 mL) warm water. Set aside for 5 minutes. Add with the liquids. You may need to increase the baking time by 5 to 10 minutes.

Variation

For an even tangier taste, add 1 tsp (5 mL) vinegar with the liquids.

Sourdough Loaf
(Bread Machine Method)

Makes 15 slices (1 per serving)

Try this warm creamy loaf the next time you feel like eating a sandwich.

Tip

To ensure success, see page 174 for extra information on baking yeast bread in a bread machine and read "Tips for Successful Starters," page 201.

1 cup	brown rice flour	250 mL
1 cup	amaranth flour	250 mL
½ cup	potato starch	125 mL
2 tbsp	granulated sugar	25 mL
1 tbsp	xanthan gum	15 mL
1 tbsp	bread machine or instant yeast	15 mL
1½ tsp	salt	7 mL
1 cup	Sourdough Starter (see recipe, page 200), at room temperature	250 mL
¼ cup	water	50 mL
¼ cup	vegetable oil	50 mL
2	eggs, lightly beaten	2
2	egg whites, lightly beaten	2

1. In a large bowl or plastic bag, combine brown rice flour, amaranth flour, potato starch, sugar, xanthan gum, yeast and salt. Mix well and set aside.

2. Pour sourdough starter, water and oil into the bread machine baking pan. Add eggs and egg whites.

3. Select the **Dough Cycle**. As the bread machine is mixing, gradually add the dry ingredients, scraping bottom and sides of pan with a rubber spatula. Try to incorporate all the dry ingredients within 1 to 2 minutes. When the mixing and kneading are complete, remove the kneading blade, leaving the bread pan in the bread machine. Quickly smooth the top of the loaf. Allow the cycle to finish. Turn off the bread machine.

4. Select the **Bake Cycle**. Set time to 60 minutes and temperature to 350°F (180°C). Allow the cycle to finish. Remove loaf from the pan immediately and let cool completely on a rack.

NUTRITIONAL VALUE
per serving

Calories	171
Fat, total	5 g
Fat, saturated	1 g
Cholesterol	25 mg
Sodium	250 mg
Carbohydrate	27 g
Fiber	3 g
Protein	5 g
Calcium	19 mg
Iron	3 mg

Variation

For an even tangier taste, add 1 tsp (5 mL) vinegar with the liquids.

Sourdough Walnut Bread
(Bread Machine Method)

Makes 15 slices (1 per serving)

We have adapted this loaf from a traditional French Canadian sourdough hearth bread.

Tip

To ensure success, see page 174 for extra information on baking yeast bread in a bread machine and read "Tips for Successful Starters," page 201.

1¼ cups	amaranth flour	300 mL
½ cup	quinoa flour	125 mL
½ cup	tapioca starch	125 mL
¼ cup	packed brown sugar	50 mL
1 tbsp	xanthan gum	15 mL
1½ tsp	bread machine or instant yeast	7 mL
1¼ tsp	salt	6 mL
1 cup	chopped walnuts	250 mL
1 cup	Sourdough Starter (see recipe, page 200), at room temperature	250 mL
⅔ cup	water	150 mL
2 tbsp	vegetable oil	25 mL
2	eggs, lightly beaten	2

1. In a large bowl or plastic bag, combine amaranth flour, quinoa flour, tapioca starch, brown sugar, xanthan gum, yeast, salt and walnuts. Mix well and set aside.

2. Pour sourdough starter, water and oil into the bread machine baking pan. Add eggs.

3. Select the **Dough Cycle**. As the bread machine is mixing, gradually add the dry ingredients, scraping bottom and sides of pan with a rubber spatula. Try to incorporate all the dry ingredients within 1 to 2 minutes. When the mixing and kneading are complete, remove the kneading blade, leaving the bread pan in the bread machine. Quickly smooth the top of the loaf. Allow the cycle to finish. Turn off the bread machine.

4. Select **Bake Cycle**. Set time to 60 minutes and temperature to 350°F (180°C). Allow the cycle to finish. Remove loaf from the pan immediately and let cool completely on a rack.

NUTRITIONAL VALUE per serving

Calories	197
Fat, total	9 g
Fat, saturated	1 g
Cholesterol	25 mg
Sodium	206 mg
Carbohydrate	26 g
Fiber	3 g
Protein	5 g
Calcium	34 mg
Iron	4 mg

Variation

For an even tangier taste, add 1 tsp (5 mL) vinegar with the liquids.

Sourdough Walnut Bread
(Mixer Method)

We have adapted this loaf from a traditional French Canadian sourdough hearth bread.

Tips

To ensure success, see page 175 for extra information on baking yeast bread using the mixer method and read "Tips for Successful Starters," page 201.

♦

Don't forget about the sourdough starter sitting in your refrigerator. If you haven't used it to make a loaf in the last 10 days, see page 201 for information on feeding it.

 9- by 5- inch (2 L) loaf pan, lightly greased

1 cup	amaranth flour	250 mL
½ cup	quinoa flour	125 mL
⅓ cup	tapioca starch	75 mL
¼ cup	packed brown sugar	50 mL
1 tbsp	xanthan gum	15 mL
1½ tsp	bread machine or instant yeast	7 mL
1¼ tsp	salt	6 mL
¾ cup	chopped walnuts	175 mL
2	eggs	2
1 cup	Sourdough Starter (see recipe, page 200), at room temperature	250 mL
½ cup	water	125 mL
2 tbsp	vegetable oil	25 mL

1. In a large bowl or plastic bag, combine amaranth flour, quinoa flour, tapioca starch, brown sugar, xanthan gum, yeast, salt and walnuts. Mix well and set aside.

2. In a separate bowl, using a heavy-duty electric mixer with paddle attachment, combine eggs, sourdough starter, water and oil until well blended. With the mixer on its lowest speed, slowly add the dry ingredients until combined. Stop the machine and scrape the bottom and sides of the bowl with a rubber spatula. With the mixer on medium speed, beat for 4 minutes.

3. Spoon into prepared pan. Let rise, uncovered, in a warm, draft-free place for 60 to 80 minutes, or until dough has risen to the top of the pan. Meanwhile, preheat oven to 350°F (180°C).

4. Bake for 35 to 45 minutes, tenting with foil partway through, or until loaf sounds hollow when tapped on the bottom. Remove from the pan immediately and let cool completely on a rack.

NUTRITIONAL VALUE per serving	
Calories	172
Fat, total	7 g
Fat, saturated	1 g
Cholesterol	25 mg
Sodium	205 mg
Carbohydrate	23 g
Fiber	3 g
Protein	5 g
Calcium	29 mg
Iron	3 mg

Tip

Tent with foil partway through the baking time, as this is a very dark-colored loaf.

To make this recipe egg-free

Omit eggs from the recipe. Combine $\frac{1}{3}$ cup (75 mL) flax flour or ground flaxseed with an additional $\frac{1}{2}$ cup (125 mL) warm water. Set aside for 5 minutes. Add with the liquids. You may need to increase the baking time by 5 to 10 minutes.

Variation

For an even tangier taste, add 1 tsp (5 mL) vinegar with the liquids.

Sourdough Brown Bread
(Mixer Method)

**Makes 15 slices
(1 per serving)**

This dense, moist, tangy bread makes wonderful sandwich bread or breakfast toast.

Tips

To ensure success, see page 175 for extra information on baking yeast bread using the mixer method and read "Tips for Successful Starters," page 201.

Don't forget about the sourdough starter sitting in your refrigerator. If you haven't used it to make a loaf in the last 10 days, see page 201 for information on feeding it.

NUTRITIONAL VALUE per serving	
Calories	121
Fat, total	3 g
Fat, saturated	0 g
Cholesterol	25 mg
Sodium	203 mg
Carbohydrate	21 g
Fiber	2 g
Protein	4 g
Calcium	12 mg
Iron	1 mg

◆ *9- by 5-inch (2 L) loaf pan, lightly greased*

1 cup	sorghum flour	250 mL
½ cup	whole bean flour	125 mL
⅓ cup	tapioca starch	75 mL
1 tbsp	xanthan gum	15 mL
1 tbsp	bread machine or instant yeast	15 mL
1¼ tsp	salt	6 mL
2	eggs	2
1 cup	Sourdough Starter (see recipe, page 200), at room temperature	250 mL
½ cup	water	125 mL
2 tbsp	vegetable oil	25 mL
2 tbsp	liquid honey	25 mL
1 tbsp	fancy molasses	15 mL

1. In a large bowl or plastic bag, combine sorghum flour, whole bean flour, tapioca starch, xanthan gum, yeast and salt. Mix well and set aside.

2. In a separate bowl, using a heavy-duty electric mixer with paddle attachment, combine eggs, sourdough starter, water, oil, honey and molasses until well blended. With the mixer on its lowest speed, slowly add the dry ingredients until combined. Stop the machine and scrape the bottom and sides of the bowl with a rubber spatula. With the mixer on medium speed, beat for 4 minutes.

3. Spoon into prepared pan. Let rise, uncovered, in a warm, draft-free place for 60 to 80 minutes, or until dough has risen to the top of the pan. Meanwhile, preheat oven to 350°F (180°C).

4. Bake for 35 to 45 minutes, or until loaf sounds hollow when tapped on the bottom. Remove from the pan immediately and let cool completely on a rack.

Tip

It is easier to measure honey and molasses if they are warmed in the microwave for a few seconds, or set in a pan of hot water for a few minutes. Measure the oil first, then measure the honey and molasses; they will slide off the measuring spoon more easily that way.

To make this recipe egg-free

Omit eggs from the recipe. Combine $\frac{1}{3}$ cup (75 mL) flax flour or ground flaxseed with an additional $\frac{1}{3}$ cup (75 mL) warm water. Set aside for 5 minutes. Add with the liquids. You may need to increase the baking time by 5 to 10 minutes.

Variations

Substitute $\frac{1}{4}$ cup (50 mL) packed brown sugar for the honey and the molasses.

For an even tangier taste, add 1 tsp (5 mL) cider vinegar with the liquids.

Sourdough Brown Bread
(Bread Machine Method)

Makes 15 slices (1 per serving)

This dense, moist, tangy bread makes wonderful sandwich bread or breakfast toast.

Tips

To ensure success, see page 174 for extra information on baking yeast bread in a bread machine and read "Tips for Successful Starters," page 201.

Don't forget about the sourdough starter sitting in your refrigerator. If you haven't used it to make a loaf in the last 10 days, see page 201 for information on feeding it.

1 cup	sorghum flour	250 mL
⅔ cup	whole bean flour	150 mL
⅓ cup	tapioca starch	75 mL
1 tbsp	xanthan gum	15 mL
1 tbsp	bread machine or instant yeast	15 mL
1¼ tsp	salt	6 mL
1 cup	Sourdough Starter (see recipe, page 200), at room temperature	250 mL
¾ cup	water	175 mL
2 tbsp	vegetable oil	25 mL
2 tbsp	liquid honey	25 mL
2 tbsp	fancy molasses	25 mL
2	eggs, lightly beaten	2

1. In a large bowl or plastic bag, combine sorghum flour, whole bean flour, tapioca starch, xanthan gum, yeast and salt. Mix well and set aside.

2. Pour sourdough starter, water, oil, honey and molasses into the bread machine baking pan. Add eggs.

3. Select the **Dough Cycle**. As the bread machine is mixing, gradually add the dry ingredients, scraping bottom and sides of pan with a rubber spatula. Try to incorporate all the dry ingredients within 1 to 2 minutes. When the mixing and kneading are complete, remove the kneading blade, leaving the bread pan in the bread machine. Quickly smooth the top of the loaf. Allow the cycle to finish. Turn off the bread machine.

4. Select the **Bake Cycle**. Set time to 60 minutes and temperature to 350°F (180°C). Allow the cycle to finish. Remove loaf from the pan immediately and let cool completely on a rack.

NUTRITIONAL VALUE per serving	
Calories	131
Fat, total	3 g
Fat, saturated	0 g
Cholesterol	25 mg
Sodium	204 mg
Carbohydrate	23 g
Fiber	2 g
Protein	4 g
Calcium	19 mg
Iron	1 mg

Tip

It is easier to measure honey and molasses if they are warmed in the microwave for a few seconds, or set in a pan of hot water for a few minutes. Measure the oil first, then measure the honey and molasses; they will slide off the measuring spoon more easily that way.

To make this recipe egg-free
Omit eggs from the recipe. Combine ⅓ cup (75 mL) flax flour or ground flaxseed with an additional ⅓ cup (75 mL) warm water. Set aside for 5 minutes. Add with the liquids.

Variations

Substitute ¼ cup (50 mL) packed brown sugar for the honey and the molasses.

For an even tangier taste, add 1 tsp (5 mL) cider vinegar with the liquids.

Sourdough Savory Ciabatta

Makes 8 wedges (1 per serving)

The name "ciabatta" refers to the traditional slipper shape. We've adapted the shape to accommodate the batter-like gluten-free dough. This version has a designer twist for those who like their yeast breads tangy and sour.

Tips

To ensure success, see pages 174–175 for extra information on baking yeast bread in a bread machine or using the mixer method and read "Tips for Successful Starters," page 201.

We like this ciabatta best served hot out of the oven.

NUTRITIONAL VALUE per serving

Calories	198
Fat, total	6 g
Fat, saturated	1 g
Cholesterol	47 mg
Sodium	164 mg
Carbohydrate	31 g
Fiber	5 g
Protein	7 g
Calcium	73 mg
Iron	5 mg

♦ 8-inch (20 cm), round baking pan, lightly greased and floured with sweet rice flour

½ cup	amaranth flour	125 mL
⅓ cup	sorghum flour	75 mL
¼ cup	tapioca starch	50 mL
1 tbsp	granulated sugar	15 mL
2 tsp	xanthan gum	10 mL
2 tbsp	bread machine or instant yeast	25 mL
½ tsp	salt	2 mL
¼ cup	chopped fresh savory	50 mL
1 cup	Sourdough Starter (see recipe, page 200), at room temperature	250 mL
¼ cup	water	50 mL
2 tbsp	extra-virgin olive oil	25 mL
2	eggs, lightly beaten	2
2 to 3 tbsp	sweet rice flour, brown rice flour or sorghum flour	25 to 45 mL

Bread Machine Method

1. In a large bowl or plastic bag, combine amaranth flour, sorghum flour, tapioca starch, sugar, xanthan gum, yeast, salt and savory. Mix well and set aside.

2. Pour sourdough starter, water and olive oil into the bread machine baking pan. Add eggs. Select the **Dough Cycle**. As the bread machine is mixing, gradually add the dry ingredients, scraping bottom and sides of pan with a rubber spatula. Try to incorporate all the dry ingredients within 1 to 2 minutes. Stop bread machine as soon as the kneading portion of the cycle is complete. Do not let bread machine finish the cycle.

Mixer Method

1. In a large bowl or plastic bag, combine amaranth flour, sorghum flour, tapioca starch, sugar, xanthan gum, yeast, salt and savory. Mix well and set aside.

Tips

Break this bread into pieces to serve with soups or salads.

A silicone baking pan works well for this recipe.

2. In a separate bowl, using a heavy-duty electric mixer with paddle attachment, combine sourdough starter, water, olive oil and eggs until well blended. With the mixer on its lowest speed, slowly add the dry ingredients until combined. Stop the machine and scrape the bottom and sides of the bowl with a rubber spatula. With the mixer on medium speed, beat for 4 minutes.

For Both Methods

3. Immediately transfer dough to prepared pan and spread evenly. Generously dust top with sweet rice flour. With well-floured fingers, make deep indents all over the dough, making sure to press all the way down to the pan. Let rise, uncovered, in a warm, draft-free place for 45 to 60 minutes, or until almost double in volume. Meanwhile, preheat oven to 425°F (220°C).

4. Bake for 18 to 20 minutes, or until bread is golden and sounds hollow when top is tapped. Remove from the pan immediately. Cut into 8 wedges and serve hot.

To make this recipe egg-free

Omit eggs from the recipe. Combine ⅓ cup (75 mL) flax flour or ground flaxseed with an additional ¼ cup (50 mL) warm water. Set aside for 5 minutes. Add with liquid ingredients. If using the mixer method, you may need to increase the baking time by 5 to 10 minutes.

Variations

If fresh savory is not available, use one-third the amount of dried savory. Or substitute an equal amount of your favorite herb — rosemary, thyme or cilantro work well, to name a few.

For a thinner ciabatta, bake in a 9-inch (23 cm) round baking pan and increase the baking time to 21 minutes.

Olive Ciabatta

Makes 8 wedges (1 per serving)

Black and green olives and a good-quality olive oil combine to make this strong-flavored, irresistible Italian bread. We've adapted the shape to accommodate the batter-like gluten-free dough.

Tips

To ensure success, see pages 174–175 for extra information on baking yeast bread in a bread machine or using the mixer method.

Be sure olives are well drained and pat dry with paper towels.

◆ 8-inch (20 cm) round baking pan, lightly greased

½ cup	hazelnut flour	125 mL
½ cup	whole bean flour	125 mL
¼ cup	quinoa flour	50 mL
¼ cup	tapioca starch	50 mL
2 tbsp	granulated sugar	25 mL
2 tsp	xanthan gum	10 mL
1 tbsp	bread machine or instant yeast	15 mL
1 tsp	salt	5 mL
1 tbsp	dried oregano	15 mL
1 tbsp	dried rosemary	15 mL
¾ cup	water	175 mL
2 tbsp	extra-virgin olive oil	25 mL
1 tsp	cider vinegar	5 mL
2	eggs, lightly beaten	2
¾ cup	pitted sliced Kalamata olives	175 mL
¾ cup	pitted sliced green olives	175 mL
½ cup	chopped hazelnuts	125 mL
2 to 3 tbsp	sweet rice flour, brown rice flour or whole bean flour	25 to 45 mL

Bread Machine Method

1. In a large bowl or plastic bag, combine hazelnut flour, whole bean flour, quinoa flour, tapioca starch, sugar, xanthan gum, yeast, salt, oregano and rosemary. Mix well and set aside.

2. Pour water, olive oil and vinegar into the bread machine baking pan. Add eggs. Select the **Dough Cycle**. As the bread machine is mixing, gradually add the dry ingredients, scraping bottom and sides of pan with a rubber spatula. Try to incorporate all the dry ingredients within 1 to 2 minutes. Stop bread machine as soon as the kneading portion of the cycle is complete. Do not let bread machine finish the cycle. Remove baking pan from the bread machine. Fold in Kalamata olives, green olives and hazelnuts.

NUTRITIONAL VALUE per serving

Calories	238
Fat, total	16 g
Fat, saturated	2 g
Cholesterol	47 mg
Sodium	611 mg
Carbohydrate	19 g
Fiber	4 g
Protein	6 g
Calcium	55 mg
Iron	2 mg

Tips

When dusting with sweet rice flour, use a flour sifter for a light, even sprinkle.

If you'd prefer to make 4 to 6 individual ciabatta, use English muffin rings and fill two-thirds full.

Mixer Method

1. In a large bowl or plastic bag, combine hazelnut flour, whole bean flour, quinoa flour, tapioca starch, sugar, xanthan gum, yeast, salt, oregano and rosemary. Mix well and set aside.

2. In a separate bowl, using a heavy-duty electric mixer with paddle attachment, combine water, olive oil, vinegar and eggs until well blended. With the mixer on its lowest speed, slowly add the dry ingredients until combined. Stop the machine and scrape the bottom and sides of the bowl with a rubber spatula. With the mixer on medium speed, beat for 4 minutes. Fold in Kalamata olives, green olives and hazelnuts.

For Both Methods

3. Gently transfer dough to prepared pan and spread evenly to the edges, leaving the top rough and uneven. Generously dust top with sweet rice flour. With well-floured fingers, make deep indents all over the dough, making sure to press all the way down to the pan. Let rise, uncovered, in a warm, draft-free place for 60 to 75 minutes, or until almost double in volume. Meanwhile, preheat oven to 400°F (200°C).

4. Bake for 20 to 25 minutes, or until top is golden. Remove from the pan immediately. Cut into 8 wedges.

To make this recipe egg-free
Omit eggs from the recipe. Combine $1/2$ cup (125 mL) flax flour or ground flaxseed with an additional $1/4$ cup (50 mL) warm water. Set aside for 5 minutes. Add with the liquids. If using the mixer method, you may need to increase the baking time by 5 to 10 minutes.

Variation

To turn this into a Mediterranean-style ciabatta, add $1/2$ cup (125 mL) finely chopped red onion with the Kalamata olives and substitute 1 tbsp (15 mL) snipped fresh cilantro or mint for the green olives.

Honey Dijon Toastie

Makes 10 wedges (1 per serving)

A small amount of honey mustard added to the dough makes this open-textured bread an ideal sandwich bread (see Barbecued Tuscan Toastie, page 88) or accompaniment to a baked ham dinner.

Tip

To ensure success, see pages 174–175 for extra information on baking yeast bread in a bread machine or using the mixer method.

♦ *9-inch (23 cm) round baking pan, lightly greased*

1¼ cups	whole bean flour	300 mL
¼ cup	quinoa flour	50 mL
⅓ cup	tapioca starch	75 mL
2 tsp	xanthan gum	10 mL
2 tbsp	bread machine or instant yeast	25 mL
¼ tsp	salt	1 mL
2 tsp	dried thyme	10 mL
1¾ cups	water	425 mL
¼ cup	extra-virgin olive oil	50 mL
¼ cup	liquid honey	50 mL
1 tsp	cider vinegar	5 mL
¼ cup	honey Dijon mustard	50 mL
2	cloves garlic, minced	2

Bread Machine Method

1. In a large bowl or plastic bag, combine whole bean flour, quinoa flour, tapioca starch, xanthan gum, yeast, salt and thyme. Mix well and set aside.

2. Pour water, olive oil, honey, vinegar, mustard and garlic into the bread machine baking pan. Select the **Dough Cycle**. As the bread machine is mixing, gradually add the dry ingredients, scraping bottom and sides of pan with a rubber spatula. Try to incorporate all the dry ingredients within 1 to 2 minutes. Stop bread machine as soon as the kneading portion of the cycle is complete. Do not let bread machine finish cycle.

Mixer Method

1. In a large bowl or plastic bag, combine whole bean flour, quinoa flour, tapioca starch, xanthan gum, yeast, salt and thyme. Mix well and set aside.

NUTRITIONAL VALUE per serving

Calories	146
Fat, total	6 g
Fat, saturated	1 g
Cholesterol	0 mg
Sodium	151 mg
Carbohydrate	20 g
Fiber	1 g
Protein	3 g
Calcium	18 mg
Iron	1 mg

2. In a separate bowl, using a heavy-duty electric mixer with paddle attachment, combine water, olive oil, honey, vinegar, mustard and garlic until well blended. With the mixer on its lowest speed, slowly add the dry ingredients until combined. Stop the machine and scrape the bottom and sides of the bowl with a rubber spatula. With the mixer on medium speed, beat for 4 minutes.

For Both Methods

3. Gently transfer dough to prepared pan and spread evenly. With wet fingers, make deep indents all over the dough, making sure to press all the way down to the pan. Let rise, uncovered, in a warm, draft-free place for 30 to 45 minutes, or until almost to the top of pan. Meanwhile, preheat oven to 375°F (190°C).

4. Bake for 18 to 25 minutes, or until top is golden. Remove from the pan immediately and serve hot or transfer to a cooling rack and let cool completely.

Variation

Add 2 to 3 tsp (10 to 15 mL) dried herbs to the soft dough, then sprinkle with 2 to 3 tbsp (25 to 45 mL) freshly grated lactose-free Parmesan cheese or Parmesan cheese before making indents with wet fingers.

Pizza Crust

**Makes 6 pieces,
each 5 by 5 inches
(12.5 by 12.5 cm)
(1 per serving)**

Use this thin crust to
make Florentine Pizza
(page 86) or Sausage and
Leek Pizza (page 87).

Tip

To ensure success, see
pages 174–175 for extra
information on baking
yeast bread in a bread
machine or using the
mixer method.

♦ *Preheat oven to 400°F (200°C)*
♦ *15- by 10-inch (40 by 25 cm) jelly-roll pan, lightly greased*

⅔ cup	sorghum flour	150 mL
½ cup	quinoa flour	125 mL
⅓ cup	potato starch	75 mL
¼ cup	tapioca starch	50 mL
1 tsp	granulated sugar	5 mL
2 tsp	xanthan gum	10 mL
1 tbsp	bread machine or instant yeast	15 mL
¾ tsp	salt	4 mL
1¼ cups	water	300 mL
1 tbsp	extra-virgin olive oil	15 mL
1 tsp	cider vinegar	5 mL

Bread Machine Method

1. In a large bowl or plastic bag, combine sorghum flour,
quinoa flour, potato starch, tapioca starch, sugar,
xanthan gum, yeast and salt. Mix well and set aside.

2. Pour water, olive oil and vinegar into the bread
machine baking pan. Select the **Dough Cycle**. As
the bread machine is mixing, gradually add the dry
ingredients, scraping bottom and sides of pan with
a rubber spatula. Try to incorporate all the dry
ingredients within 1 to 2 minutes. Stop bread
machine as soon as the kneading portion of the cycle
is complete. Do not let bread machine finish the cycle.

Mixer Method

1. In a large bowl or plastic bag, combine sorghum flour,
quinoa flour, potato starch, tapioca starch, sugar,
xanthan gum, yeast and salt. Mix well and set aside.

2. In a separate bowl, using a heavy-duty electric mixer
with paddle attachment, combine water, olive oil and
vinegar until well blended. With the mixer on lowest
speed, slowly add the dry ingredients until combined.
Stop the machine and scrape the bottom and sides of
the bowl with a rubber spatula. With the mixer on
medium speed, beat for 4 minutes.

Partially baked pizza crust can be wrapped airtight and frozen for up to 4 weeks. Thaw in the refrigerator overnight before using to make pizza.

For Both Methods

3. Gently transfer the dough to prepared pan and spread evenly to the edges. Do not smooth top.

4. Bake in preheated oven for 12 minutes, or until bottom is golden and crust is partially baked.

Variations

Add 1 to 2 tsp (5 to 10 mL) dried or 1 to 2 tbsp (15 to 25 mL) chopped fresh rosemary, oregano, basil or thyme to the dry ingredients.

To make individual pizzas, divide dough into 4 equal portions and pat into 6-inch (15 cm) diameter circles. Bake on greased baking sheets for 10 to 12 minutes before adding toppings. After adding toppings, bake for an additional 10 to 12 minutes.

Rich Dinner Rolls

Makes 6 rolls (1 per serving)

This is the answer to a special request for a recipe to make just a half-dozen everyday dinner rolls.

Tip

To ensure success, see pages 174–175 for extra information on baking yeast bread in a bread machine or using the mixer method.

♦ *6-cup muffin tin, lightly greased*

½ cup	almond flour	125 mL
½ cup	brown rice flour	125 mL
¼ cup	amaranth flour	50 mL
¼ cup	potato starch	50 mL
2 tsp	xanthan gum	10 mL
1¾ tsp	bread machine or instant yeast	8 mL
¾ tsp	salt	4 mL
¾ cup	lactose-free plain yogurt or plain yogurt	175 mL
2 tbsp	vegetable oil	25 mL
2 tbsp	liquid honey	25 mL
1	egg, lightly beaten	1
1	egg white, lightly beaten	1

Bread Machine Method

1. In a large bowl or plastic bag, combine almond flour, brown rice flour, amaranth flour, potato starch, xanthan gum, yeast and salt. Mix well and set aside.

2. Pour yogurt, oil and honey into the bread machine baking pan. Add egg and egg white. Select the **Dough Cycle**. As the bread machine is mixing, gradually add the dry ingredients, scraping bottom and sides of pan with a rubber spatula. Try to incorporate all the dry ingredients within 1 to 2 minutes. Stop bread machine as soon as the kneading portion of the cycle is complete. Do not let bread machine finish the cycle.

Mixer Method

1. In a large bowl or plastic bag, combine almond flour, brown rice flour, amaranth flour, potato starch, xanthan gum, yeast and salt. Mix well and set aside.

2. In a separate bowl, using a heavy-duty electric mixer with paddle attachment, combine yogurt, oil, honey, egg and egg white until well blended. With the mixer on its lowest speed, slowly add the dry ingredients until combined. Stop the machine and scrape the bottom and sides of the bowl with a rubber spatula. With the mixer on medium speed, beat for 4 minutes.

NUTRITIONAL VALUE per serving

Calories	243
Fat, total	11 g
Fat, saturated	1 g
Cholesterol	31 mg
Sodium	323 mg
Carbohydrate	29 g
Fiber	3 g
Protein	7 g
Calcium	44 mg
Iron	3 mg

For Both Methods

3. Using a $\frac{1}{4}$-cup (50 mL) scoop, divide dough into 6 equal amounts and place in cups of prepared muffin tin. Let rise, uncovered, in a warm, draft-free place for 60 minutes. Meanwhile, preheat oven to 400°F (200°C).

4. Bake for 18 to 20 minutes, or until rolls sound hollow when tapped on the bottom. Remove from the pan immediately and let cool completely on a rack.

To make this recipe egg-free

Omit egg and egg white from the recipe. Add 1 tbsp (15 mL) powdered egg replacer with the dry ingredients and add $\frac{1}{4}$ cup (50 mL) of water with the yogurt. If using the mixer method, you may need to increase the baking time by 5 to 10 minutes.

Variation

To make a dozen dinner rolls, double the ingredients, except for the xanthan gum and the yeast.

Brown Seed Dinner Rolls

Makes 12 rolls (1 per serving)

Longing for a rich, dark dinner roll? We've added three kinds of seeds for extra crunch.

Tip

To ensure success, see pages 174–175 for extra information on baking yeast bread in a bread machine or using the mixer method.

♦ *12-cup muffin tin, lightly greased*

¾ cup	sorghum flour	175 mL
¾ cup	whole bean flour	175 mL
¼ cup	potato starch	50 mL
¼ cup	rice bran	50 mL
2½ tsp	xanthan gum	12 mL
1 tbsp	bread machine or instant yeast	15 mL
1¼ tsp	salt	6 mL
⅓ cup	green pumpkin seeds	75 mL
⅓ cup	raw unsalted sunflower seeds	75 mL
¼ cup	sesame seeds	50 mL
1¼ cups	water	300 mL
¼ cup	vegetable oil	50 mL
2 tbsp	liquid honey	25 mL
2 tbsp	fancy molasses	25 mL
1 tsp	cider vinegar	5 mL
2	eggs, lightly beaten	2

Bread Machine Method

1. In a large bowl or plastic bag, combine sorghum flour, whole bean flour, potato starch, rice bran, xanthan gum, yeast, salt, pumpkin seeds, sunflower seeds and sesame seeds. Mix well and set aside.

2. Pour water, oil, honey, molasses and vinegar into the bread machine baking pan. Add eggs. Select the **Dough Cycle**. As the bread machine is mixing, gradually add the dry ingredients, scraping bottom and sides of pan with a rubber spatula. Try to incorporate all the dry ingredients within 1 to 2 minutes. Stop bread machine as soon as the kneading portion of the cycle is complete. Do not let bread machine finish the cycle.

Mixer Method

1. In a large bowl or plastic bag, combine sorghum flour, whole bean flour, potato starch, rice bran, xanthan gum, yeast, salt, pumpkin seeds, sunflower seeds and sesame seeds. Mix well and set aside.

NUTRITIONAL VALUE per serving

Calories	192
Fat, total	11 g
Fat, saturated	1 g
Cholesterol	31 mg
Sodium	256 mg
Carbohydrate	20 g
Fiber	3 g
Protein	6 g
Calcium	56 mg
Iron	3 mg

If you don't have a scoop, use a large serving spoon and drop into muffin cups by large rounded spoonfuls.

2. In a separate bowl, using a heavy-duty electric mixer with paddle attachment, combine water, oil, honey, molasses, vinegar and eggs until well blended. With the mixer on its lowest speed, slowly add the dry ingredients until combined. Stop the machine and scrape the bottom and sides of the bowl with a rubber spatula. With the mixer on medium speed, beat for 4 minutes.

For Both Methods

3. Using a $\frac{1}{4}$-cup (50 mL) scoop, divide dough into 12 equal amounts and place in cups of prepared muffin tin. Let rise, uncovered, in a warm, draft-free place for 60 minutes. Meanwhile, preheat oven to 350°F (180°C).

4. Bake for 18 to 20 minutes, or until rolls sound hollow when tapped on the bottom. Remove from the pan immediately and let cool completely on a rack.

To make this recipe egg-free
Omit eggs from the recipe. Combine $\frac{1}{3}$ cup (75 mL) flax flour or ground flaxseed with an additional $\frac{1}{4}$ cup (50 mL) warm water. Set aside for 5 minutes. Add with the liquids. If using the mixer method, you may need to increase the baking time by 5 to 10 minutes.

Variations

Instead of using a muffin tin, drop 12 spoonfuls of dough at least 2 inches (5 cm) apart onto a lightly greased baking sheet.

Before letting dough rise, sprinkle tops with $\frac{1}{4}$ cup (50 mL) sesame seeds. The seeds will toast as the rolls bake.

Bread Sticks

Serve these bread sticks
as Italian restaurants
do — with a dish of
flavored olive oil for
dipping.

Tips

To ensure success, see
pages 174–175 for extra
information on baking
yeast bread in a bread
machine or using the
mixer method.

Thoroughly mix the dry
ingredients before adding
them to the liquids —
they are powder-fine and
can clump together.

To make your own
almond flour, see under
Nut flour in the
Technique Glossary,
page 301.

**NUTRITIONAL VALUE
per serving**

Calories	82
Fat, total	3 g
Fat, saturated	0 g
Cholesterol	0 mg
Sodium	148 mg
Carbohydrate	12 g
Fiber	1 g
Protein	2 g
Calcium	27 mg
Iron	1 mg

- *9-inch (2.5 L) square baking pan, lightly greased*
- *Baking sheet, ungreased*

⅔ cup	brown rice flour	150 mL
2 tbsp	almond flour	25 mL
¼ cup	potato starch	50 mL
2 tbsp	tapioca starch	25 mL
1 tbsp	granulated sugar	15 mL
1¼ tsp	xanthan gum	6 mL
2 tsp	bread machine or instant yeast	10 mL
¾ tsp	salt	4 mL
¾ cup	water	175 mL
1 tbsp	vegetable oil	15 mL
1 tsp	cider vinegar	5 mL
3 tbsp	sesame seeds	45 mL

Bread Machine Method

1. In a large bowl or plastic bag, combine brown rice flour, almond flour, potato starch, tapioca starch, sugar, xanthan gum, yeast and salt. Mix well and set aside.

2. Pour water, oil and vinegar into the bread machine baking pan. Select the **Dough Cycle**. As the bread machine is mixing, gradually add the dry ingredients, scraping bottom and sides of pan with a rubber spatula. Try to incorporate all the dry ingredients within 1 to 2 minutes. Stop bread machine as soon as the kneading portion of the cycle is complete. Do not let bread machine finish the cycle.

Mixer Method

1. In a large bowl or plastic bag, combine brown rice flour, almond flour, potato starch, tapioca starch, sugar, xanthan gum, yeast and salt. Mix well and set aside.

2. In a separate bowl, using a heavy-duty electric mixer with paddle attachment, combine water, oil and vinegar until well blended. With the mixer on its lowest speed, slowly add the dry ingredients until combined. Stop the machine and scrape the bottom and sides of the bowl with a rubber spatula. With the mixer on medium speed, beat for 4 minutes.

Tips

Don't worry when seeds move as you spread the dough to the edges of the pan — they will still coat the bread sticks.

For uniform bread sticks, cut bread in half, then lengthwise into quarters. Finally, cut each quarter lengthwise into 3 strips.

If bread sticks become soft, crisp in a toaster oven or conventional oven at 350°F (180°C) for a few minutes.

Use any leftover bread sticks to make dry bread crumbs (see the Technique Glossary, page 299).

For Both Methods

3. Sprinkle 2 tbsp (25 mL) of the sesame seeds in bottom of prepared pan. Drop dough by spoonfuls over the sesame seeds. Using a moistened rubber spatula, spread dough evenly to the edges of the pan. Sprinkle with the remaining sesame seeds. Using moistened rubber spatula, press seeds into dough. Let rise, uncovered, in a warm, draft-free place for 30 minutes. Meanwhile, preheat oven to 400°F (200°C).

4. Bake for 10 to 12 minutes, or until light brown. Remove from the pan and transfer immediately to a cutting board. Reduce oven temperature to 350°F (180°C). With a pizza wheel or a sharp knife, cut bread into 12 equal strips. Roll strips in loose sesame seeds in pan, pressing seeds into cut sides.

5. Arrange slices, with cut sides exposed, at least $\frac{1}{2}$ inch (1 cm) apart on baking sheet. Bake for 20 to 25 minutes, or until dry, crisp and golden brown. Immediately transfer to a cooling rack and let cool completely.

Variations

Substitute poppy seeds for the sesame seeds.

For an Italian herb flavor, add 2 to 3 tsp (10 to 15 mL) of your favorite dried herb with the dry ingredients and use extra-virgin olive oil instead of vegetable oil.

Stollen

Stollen is a traditional German Christmas bread with a very dark, rich-colored crust and a domed top. It is served on Christmas Eve, when families gather to celebrate before going to church.

Tip

To ensure success, see pages 174–175 for extra information on baking yeast bread in a bread machine or using the mixer method.

♦ 9-inch (23 cm) round baking pan, lightly greased

1 cup	brown rice flour	250 mL
⅓ cup	quinoa flour	75 mL
¼ cup	almond flour	50 mL
⅓ cup	arrowroot starch	75 mL
¼ cup	tapioca starch	50 mL
1 tbsp	xanthan gum	15 mL
1 tbsp	bread machine or instant yeast	15 mL
1 tsp	salt	5 mL
¾ tsp	ground cardamom	4 mL
¾ cup	chopped mixed candied fruit	175 mL
¾ cup	raisins	175 mL
1 cup	water	250 mL
3 tbsp	vegetable oil	45 mL
2	eggs, lightly beaten	2
½ cup	marmalade	125 mL

Orange Glaze

1 cup	GF confectioner's (icing) sugar, sifted	250 mL
1 to 2 tbsp	frozen orange juice concentrate, thawed	15 to 25 mL

Bread Machine Method

1. In a large bowl or plastic bag, combine brown rice flour, quinoa flour, almond flour, arrowroot starch, tapioca starch, xanthan gum, yeast, salt, cardamom, fruit and raisins. Mix well and set aside.

2. Pour water and oil into the bread machine baking pan. Add eggs and marmalade. Select the **Dough Cycle**. As the bread machine is mixing, gradually add the dry ingredients, scraping bottom and sides of pan with a rubber spatula. Try to incorporate all the dry ingredients within 1 to 2 minutes. Stop bread machine as soon as the kneading portion of the cycle is complete. Do not let bread machine finish the cycle.

NUTRITIONAL VALUE per serving	
Calories	198
Fat, total	5 g
Fat, saturated	1 g
Cholesterol	23 mg
Sodium	165 mg
Carbohydrate	37 g
Fiber	2 g
Protein	3 g
Calcium	24 mg
Iron	1 mg

Tip

Watch closely while loaf is baking — it will burn easily. You will need to tent with foil.

Mixer Method

1. In a large bowl or plastic bag, combine brown rice flour, quinoa flour, almond flour, arrowroot starch, tapioca starch, xanthan gum, yeast, salt, cardamom, fruit and raisins. Mix well and set aside.

2. In a separate bowl, using a heavy-duty electric mixer with paddle attachment, combine, water, oil, eggs and marmalade until well blended. With the mixer on its lowest speed, slowly add the dry ingredients until combined. Stop the machine and scrape the bottom and sides of the bowl with a rubber spatula. With the mixer on medium speed, beat for 4 minutes.

For Both Methods

3. Gently transfer dough to prepared pan and smooth top. Let rise, uncovered, in a warm, draft-free place for 45 minutes, or until almost to the top of pan. Meanwhile, preheat oven to 350°F (180°C).

4. Bake in bottom third of oven for 40 to 45 minutes, tenting with foil after 25 minutes, or until bread is dark golden brown and sounds hollow when top is tapped. Remove from the pan immediately and let cool completely on a rack.

5. *Prepare the orange glaze:* In a small bowl, combine confectioner's sugar and enough orange juice concentrate to make a thin glaze. Drizzle over cooled stollen.

Variation

For a more traditional presentation, omit the orange glaze and dust cooled stollen with GF confectioner's (icing) sugar to resemble a light covering of snow.

Cinnamon Buns

Makes 12 buns (1 per serving)

You asked us for a cinnamon bun you could roll out and pull apart to eat. Well, here it is! The assembly can be a bit tricky, but the dough is less sticky if kept cold.

Tips

To ensure success, see pages 174–175 for extra information on baking yeast bread in a bread machine or using the mixer method.

This dough is thicker than that of most gluten-free breads; in fact, we were able to use the dough hook attachment of the heavy-duty mixer.

NUTRITIONAL VALUE per serving

Calories	422
Fat, total	13 g
Fat, saturated	2 g
Cholesterol	31 mg
Sodium	314 mg
Carbohydrate	74 g
Fiber	5 g
Protein	7 g
Calcium	64 mg
Iron	3 mg

♦ 9-inch (23 cm) round silicone baking pan with 2-inch (5 cm) sides

1½ to 1⅔ cups	sorghum flour, divided	375 to 400 mL
¾ cup	whole bean flour	175 mL
⅔ cup	tapioca starch	150 mL
½ cup	cornstarch	125 mL
2 tbsp	potato flour (*not* potato starch)	25 mL
½ cup	granulated sugar	125 mL
1 tbsp	xanthan gum	15 mL
4 tsp	bread machine or instant yeast	20 mL
1¼ tsp	salt	6 mL
1 cup	fortified soy beverage, lactose-free milk or milk	250 mL
2 tbsp	vegetable oil	25 mL
1 tsp	cider vinegar	5 mL
2	eggs, lightly beaten	2

Pecan Pan Glaze

⅓ cup	buttery spread or butter, melted	75 mL
⅓ cup	packed brown sugar	75 mL
⅓ cup	corn syrup	75 mL
24	pecan halves	24

Raisin Pecan Filling

1½ cups	raisins	375 mL
¾ cup	chopped pecans	175 mL
⅓ cup	packed brown sugar	75 mL
⅓ cup	buttery spread or butter, softened	75 mL
1½ tsp	ground cinnamon	7 mL

Bread Machine Method

1. In a large bowl or plastic bag, combine 1 cup (250 mL) of the sorghum flour, whole bean flour, tapioca starch, cornstarch, potato flour, sugar, xanthan gum, yeast and salt. Mix well and set aside.

Tips

We don't recommend using a springform pan unless you want to clean your oven and test your smoke alarm battery — ours leaked! You can use a regular metal 9-inch (23 cm) round cake pan, as long as the sides are at least 2 inches (5 cm) high.

Be sure to prepare both the pan glaze and the filling before removing the first square of dough from the refrigerator. Work quickly when rolling out the dough and assembling the buns. Return the dough to the refrigerator for a few minutes if it becomes sticky.

We prefer to cut the dough into buns with a pizza wheel; however, kitchen shears or a sharp knife work well too. You may have to dip the cutter in hot water between cuts.

2. Pour soy beverage, oil and vinegar into the bread machine baking pan. Add eggs. Select the **Dough Cycle**. As the bread machine is mixing, gradually add the dry ingredients, scraping bottom and sides of pan with a rubber spatula. Try to incorporate all the dry ingredients within 1 to 2 minutes. Stop bread machine as soon as the kneading portion of the cycle is complete. Do not let bread machine finish the cycle.

Mixer Method

1. In a large bowl or plastic bag, combine 1 cup (250 mL) of the sorghum flour, whole bean flour, tapioca starch, cornstarch, potato flour, sugar, xanthan gum, yeast and salt. Mix well and set aside.

2. In a separate bowl, using a heavy-duty electric mixer with dough hook attachment, combine soy beverage, oil, vinegar and eggs until well blended. With the mixer on its lowest speed, slowly add the dry ingredients until combined. Stop the machine and scrape the bottom and sides of the bowl with a rubber spatula. With the mixer on medium speed, beat for 4 minutes.

For Both Methods

3. Generously coat 2 large sheets of plastic wrap with some of the remaining sorghum flour. Divide dough in half and place each half on a sheet of plastic wrap. Generously dust each with sorghum flour. Fold plastic wrap to cover dough and pat out to a square about $\frac{1}{2}$ inch (1 cm) thick. Wrap airtight and refrigerate for at least 2 hours, until chilled, or overnight.

4. *Meanwhile, prepare the pecan pan glaze:* In a small bowl, combine buttery spread, brown sugar and corn syrup. Spread evenly on bottom of pan. Arrange pecan halves, flat side up, over glaze. Set aside.

5. *Prepare the raisin pecan filling:* In a medium bowl, combine raisins, pecans, brown sugar, buttery spread and cinnamon. Set aside.

continued on next page

Tips

Freeze wrapped squares of dough for up to 1 month. Defrost overnight in the refrigerator.

Cinnamon buns can be frozen, individually wrapped, for up to 2 weeks. Defrost in the microwave.

6. Remove one square of dough from the refrigerator. Discard plastic wrap. Place on a sheet of parchment paper generously dusted with sorghum flour. Generously dust dough with sorghum flour and cover with another sheet of parchment paper. Lightly roll out to a 9-inch (23 cm) square, about ¼ inch (0.5 cm) thick. Remove top sheet of parchment paper.

7. Sprinkle half of the filling over the dough. Beginning at one side, roll up jelly-roll style, lifting the parchment paper to help the dough form a roll. With fingers, brush off excess sorghum flour. Using a pizza wheel dipped in hot water, cut into 6 equal pieces; place, cut side up, fairly close together in prepared pan. Repeat with second square of dough.

8. Let rise in a warm, draft-free place for 60 to 75 minutes, or until double in volume. Meanwhile, preheat oven to 350°F (180°C).

9. Bake for 50 to 60 minutes, tenting with foil after 40 minutes, until buns sound hollow when tapped on top. Immediately invert onto a serving platter. Let stand for 5 minutes before removing pan. Serve warm.

Variations

Substitute ¾ cup (175 mL) chopped pecans and ½ cup (125 mL) pure maple syrup or pancake syrup for the pan glaze.

Divide pecan pan glaze evenly among the cups of a lightly greased 12-cup muffin tin. Place a bun, cut side up, in each cup. Reduce baking time to 20 to 25 minutes.

A Page from Deanna's Diary

Being a youth with celiac disease can be very difficult, but I have learned that it is easier if you know other people your age with celiac disease. That way you have someone to talk to who knows exactly what you're going through. You can exchange opinions on the foods you eat and the new foods you've tried. It helps to talk about how you feel when you see your friends eating foods you can't eat and what you do to deal with those feelings. Being in contact with another celiac around your age will help you feel better about your situation, and is also a great opportunity for a lasting friendship. Meeting someone can be easy. Your local chapter of a celiac support group, such as the Canadian Celiac Association, may have a group of kids that already gets together, or you could attend a summer camp for celiac kids. Either way, it's important to make these contacts.

I've been fortunate to attend a one-week summer camp for kids with celiac disease for the past three years. It's fun to meet new kids each year and reconnect with past campers. It's great not having to worry about the food we eat, and we get lots of variety, like pizza and submarine sandwiches. At camp, we always have a self-serve buffet. This may not seem important to most people, but for celiac kids it is quite unique. We don't usually have the option to make food choices for ourselves, or to decide how much we eat. At camp we learn to make choices that include some new tastes and products, so that we can expand our day-to-day menus.

Being an adolescent with celiac disease is made much easier by having a friend with celiac disease. The companionship makes it easier to stay on the diet and helps prepare you for the challenges of eating in a world not made for you.

— Deanna Jennett, Kingston, Ontario

Authors' note: Deanna and her mother, Sue, have been celiac friends of ours since before we began developing gluten-free recipes in 2001. Deanna, now a teenager, shares her point of view in each of our gluten-free cookbooks to help other young celiacs.

Apple Butter

Makes 2½ cups (625 mL)
2 tbsp (25 mL) per serving

You won't want to wait for the crisp days of autumn to enjoy this spicy spread on everything from muffins to roast pork!

Tip

Apples that break down easily and smoothly include Empire, Gravenstein, Royal Gala, Yellow Transparent and McIntosh.

6	large apples (see tip, at left), peeled, cored and cut into eighths	6
2 cups	apple cider	500 mL
¾ cup	granulated sugar	175 mL
½ tsp	ground allspice	2 mL
½ tsp	ground cinnamon	2 mL
¼ tsp	ground cloves	1 mL

1. In a large saucepan, combine apples and apple cider. Bring to a boil over high heat. Reduce heat to medium and boil gently for 15 to 20 minutes, or until soft.
2. Transfer to a food processor fitted with a metal blade and purée until smooth.
3. Return purée to saucepan and add sugar, allspice, cinnamon and cloves. Bring to a boil over medium-high heat and cook, stirring occasionally, for 40 to 50 minutes, or until desired thickness. (Keep in mind that it will thicken more as it cools.) Store in the refrigerator for up to 2 weeks or freeze for up to 3 months.

Variations

For a more colorful apple butter, choose red-skinned apples and do not peel or core — just cut into eighths. Once tender, press through a sieve, then complete recipe. This method will give your apple butter slightly more texture. If you would like the strained butter to be smoother, transfer to a food processor and purée.

Substitute unsweetened apple juice for the apple cider.

NUTRITIONAL VALUE per serving	
Calories	65
Fat, total	0 g
Fat, saturated	0 g
Cholesterol	0 mg
Sodium	3 mg
Carbohydrate	17 g
Fiber	1 g
Protein	0 g
Calcium	4 mg
Iron	0 mg

Spicy Peach Spread

Makes 4 cups (1 L)
2 tbsp (25 mL)
per serving

When peaches are in season, purchase a basket from your local farmer's market and make this spread to serve when the season is past. It's delicious on your morning toast or layered with lactose-free plain yogurt or plain yogurt for a delightful parfait.

Tips

To quickly and easily remove peels from peaches, see the Technique Glossary, page 299, for information on blanching.

Be sure to purchase freestone peaches.

Top ham steak with Spicy Peach Spread and broil.

6	large peaches, peeled, pitted and cut into eighths	6
2 cups	peach nectar	500 mL
¼ cup	packed brown sugar	50 mL
½ tsp	ground ginger	2 mL

1. In a large saucepan, combine peaches and peach nectar. Bring to a boil over high heat. Reduce heat to medium and boil gently for 30 minutes, or until soft.

2. Transfer to a food processor fitted with a metal blade and purée until smooth.

3. Return purée to saucepan and add brown sugar and ginger. Bring to a boil over medium-low heat and cook, stirring occasionally, for 10 minutes, or until desired thickness. (Keep in mind that it will thicken more as it cools.) Store in the refrigerator for up to 2 weeks or freeze for up to 3 months.

Variation

Substitute pears for all or some of the peaches.

NUTRITIONAL VALUE per serving	
Calories	24
Fat, total	0 g
Fat, saturated	0 g
Cholesterol	0 mg
Sodium	3 mg
Carbohydrate	6 g
Fiber	1 g
Protein	0 g
Calcium	3 mg
Iron	0 mg

Pumpkin Spread

Makes 2¼ cups (550 mL)
2 tbsp (25 mL) per serving

Our friend George Hilley introduced us to this delight. We tasted it once and were hooked. Skip the butter and layer on this spread instead!

Tips

Recipe can be doubled to use a whole 28-oz (796 mL) can of pumpkin purée.

If you prefer a smoother spread, purée in a food processor or blender.

1¾ cups	canned pumpkin purée (not pie filling)	425 mL
¾ cup	unsweetened applesauce	175 mL
⅓ cup	packed brown sugar	75 mL
1 tsp	ground cinnamon	5 mL
¼ tsp	ground allspice	1 mL
¼ tsp	ground cloves	1 mL
1 tsp	freshly squeezed lemon juice	5 mL

1. In a saucepan, combine pumpkin, applesauce, brown sugar, cinnamon, allspice and cloves. Bring to a boil over medium heat, stirring constantly. Reduce heat to low and simmer gently, stirring frequently, for 5 minutes. Remove from heat and stir in lemon juice. Store in the refrigerator for up to 2 weeks or freeze for up to 3 months.

Variation

For a slightly tangier version, use apple cider instead of the applesauce.

NUTRITIONAL VALUE per serving

Calories	28
Fat, total	0 g
Fat, saturated	0 g
Cholesterol	0 mg
Sodium	3 mg
Carbohydrate	7 g
Fiber	1 g
Protein	0 g
Calcium	12 mg
Iron	1 mg

Pies and Cakes

Coconut Crust

**Makes 1 crust
(⅛ crust
per serving)**

This crust makes a great change from pastry. Fill it with banana cream (as in Banana Cream Pie, page 240), chocolate cream or coconut cream.

Tips

Only bake coconut until lightly toasted, as it continues to darken upon cooling.

Use the back of a spoon to press the coconut mixture into the pie plate, making sure it is not too thick where the sides meet the bottom.

♦ *Preheat oven to 350°F (180°C)*
♦ *9-inch (23 cm) or 8-inch (20 cm) deep-dish pie plate*

2 cups	shredded unsweetened coconut	500 mL
2 tbsp	granulated sugar	25 mL
2 tbsp	lactose-free margarine or margarine, melted	25 mL
½ tsp	grated lemon zest	2 mL

1. In a medium bowl, mix together coconut, sugar, lactose-free margarine and lemon zest until crumbly.
2. Press mixture evenly into bottom and sides of pie plate.
3. Bake in preheated oven for 10 to 12 minutes, or until lightly toasted. Let cool to room temperature before filling.

Variation
Substitute lactose-free buttery spread or butter for the lactose-free margarine or margarine.

NUTRITIONAL VALUE per serving	
Calories	152
Fat, total	14 g
Fat, saturated	8 g
Cholesterol	0 mg
Sodium	68 mg
Carbohydrate	14 g
Fiber	1 g
Protein	1 g
Calcium	4 mg
Iron	0 mg

Chocolate Walnut Crust

**Makes 1 crust
(1/10 crust
per serving)**

Not a fan of rolling out pastry? You'll love this quick, easy, no-fail crust.

Tips

The pastry is processed enough when it climbs the sides of the food processor.

Dump all the dough into the pie plate, then press evenly into the bottom and up the sides. Don't let it get too thick where the sides meet the bottom.

♦ *9-inch (23 cm) pie plate*

1 cup	walnut pieces	250 mL
½ cup	sorghum flour	125 mL
¼ cup	cornstarch	50 mL
½ tsp	xanthan gum	2 mL
¼ tsp	salt	1 mL
⅓ cup	GF confectioner's (icing) sugar, sifted	75 mL
¼ cup	unsweetened cocoa powder, sifted	50 mL
¼ cup	cold buttery spread or butter, cut into 1-inch (2.5 cm) cubes	50 mL

1. In a food processor fitted with a metal blade, pulse walnuts, sorghum flour, cornstarch, xanthan gum, salt, confectioner's sugar and cocoa 3 or 4 times to combine. Add buttery spread and pulse until mixed. Process until dough begins to hold together, scraping sides and bottom occasionally.

2. Press dough into bottom and up sides of pie plate. Cover loosely and refrigerate for at least 2 hours, until chilled, or overnight.

3. Fill and bake according to individual recipe directions or, to bake unfilled, preheat oven to 350°F (180°C). Bake for 18 to 20 minutes, or until set. Let cool completely before filling.

Variation

Use a 9-inch (23 cm) tart pan with fluted sides and a removable bottom. Place the pan on a baking sheet to make it easier to remove it from the oven. After baking, remove sides to cut wedges easily.

**NUTRITIONAL VALUE
per serving**

Calories	165
Fat, total	10 g
Fat, saturated	2 g
Cholesterol	0 mg
Sodium	85 mg
Carbohydrate	16 g
Fiber	2 g
Protein	3 g
Calcium	16 mg
Iron	1 mg

Gingerbread Crumbs

Makes 8 cups (2 L) (¼ cup/50 mL per serving)

We developed this recipe in response to the many requests we received for egg-free gingerbread crumbs. They're the perfect flavor partner for our Mango and Ginger Cream Tart (page 246) and our Lemon Cheesecake (page 254), and they make a terrific topping for parfait.

Tip

Select a shortening that is low in trans fats, if available in your area. It will not affect measuring, taste or performance.

♦ Preheat oven to 325°F (160°C)
♦ Two 15- by 10-inch (40 by 25 cm) jelly-roll pans, lightly greased

¼ cup	flax flour	50 mL
⅓ cup	warm water	75 mL
1⅔ cups	sorghum flour	400 mL
1 cup	chickpea flour	250 mL
⅓ cup	tapioca starch	75 mL
1 tsp	xanthan gum	5 mL
1 tsp	baking soda	5 mL
½ tsp	salt	2 mL
2 tsp	ground ginger	10 mL
1 tsp	ground cinnamon	5 mL
½ tsp	ground cloves	2 mL
1 cup	shortening	250 mL
¾ cup	granulated sugar	175 mL
1 cup	fancy molasses	250 mL

1. Combine flax flour and warm water. Let stand for 5 minutes.
2. Meanwhile, in a medium bowl or plastic bag, combine sorghum flour, chickpea flour, tapioca starch, xanthan gum, baking soda, salt, ginger, cinnamon and cloves; set aside.
3. In a large bowl, using an electric mixer, cream shortening, sugar, molasses and flax flour mixture until blended. Slowly beat in dry ingredients until combined.
4. Using a moistened rubber or metal spatula, spread half the batter into each prepared pan. (Remoisten spatula when the batter begins to stick to it.)
5. Bake in preheated oven for 20 minutes, or until light golden brown. Let cool completely in pans on a rack.

NUTRITIONAL VALUE per serving

Calories	148
Fat, total	7 g
Fat, saturated	1 g
Cholesterol	0 mg
Sodium	81 mg
Carbohydrate	21 g
Fiber	1 g
Protein	2 g
Calcium	32 mg
Iron	1 mg

Tips

Spread batter to an even thickness, right to the edges of the pan; this ensures that the center is cooked before the edges become too dark.

Bake both pans at the same time, in the top and bottom thirds of the oven; switch and rotate the pans halfway through the baking time.

Thaw frozen crumbs before combining with buttery spread or butter to make a crust.

6. Break gingerbread into pieces. In a food processor, working with a few pieces at a time, pulse until crumb consistency. Store in an airtight freezer bag at room temperature for up to 2 weeks or freeze for up to 3 months.

Variations

Substitute garbanzo-fava bean or whole bean (Romano) flour for the chickpea flour.

Replace the flax flour with ground flaxseed, sprouted flaxseed or Salba.

Banana Cream Pie

Makes 6 to 8 servings

Leslie Disheau and her mother, Louella Smail of Lou's Pantry in Metcalfe, Ontario, gave us the recipe for this pie filling. "It tastes great!" says Leslie. She uses a baked pie shell, but we thought you'd enjoy it in our Coconut Crust (page 236).

Tips

Drain the tofu well in a sieve; otherwise, it will not set and the filling could be watery.

Scrape down the sides of the food processor several times while puréeing the tofu.

1	package (12 oz/340 g) medium-firm silken tofu, well-drained	1
1 cup	mashed bananas	250 mL
3 tbsp	vegetable oil	45 mL
1 tsp	vanilla	5 mL
½ cup	GF confectioner's (icing) sugar, sifted	125 mL
1 tsp	freshly squeezed lemon juice	5 mL
1	banana, sliced	1
1	9-inch (23 cm) Coconut Crust, baked and cooled (see recipe, page 236)	1

1. In a food processor fitted with a metal blade, pulse tofu until smooth, scraping down sides occasionally. Add mashed bananas, oil, vanilla, confectioner's sugar and lemon juice. Pulse until smooth and creamy. Set aside.

2. Place banana slices evenly on bottom of Coconut Crust. Spoon filling over bananas. Cover loosely and refrigerate for at least 2 hours, until chilled, or overnight.

Variation

If you like a thicker layer of filling, use an 8-inch (20 cm) crust.

NUTRITIONAL VALUE
per serving

Calories	294
Fat, total	21 g
Fat, saturated	8 g
Cholesterol	0 mg
Sodium	75 mg
Carbohydrate	33 g
Fiber	2 g
Protein	4 g
Calcium	20 mg
Iron	1 mg

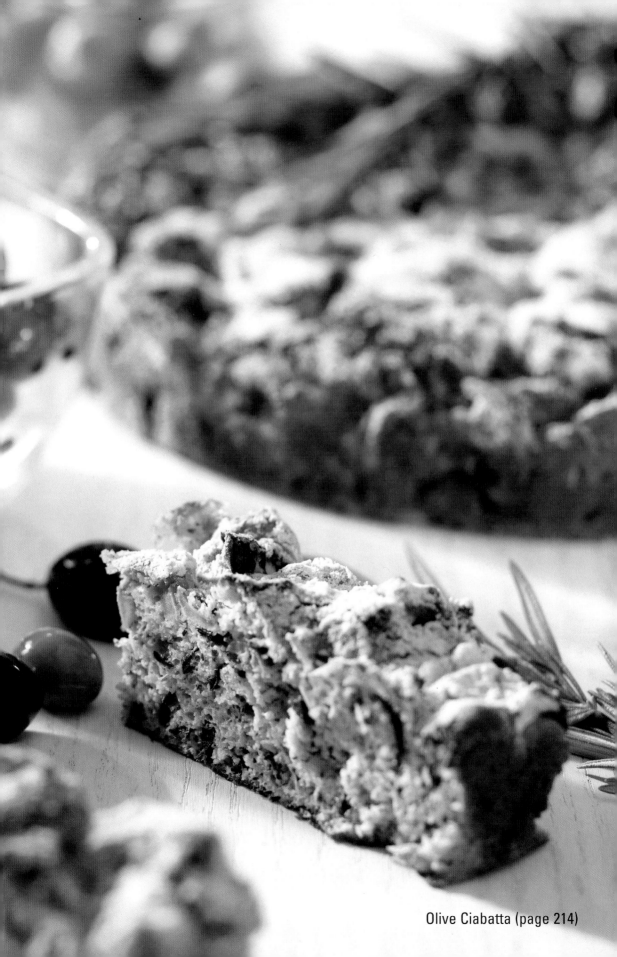

Olive Ciabatta (page 214)

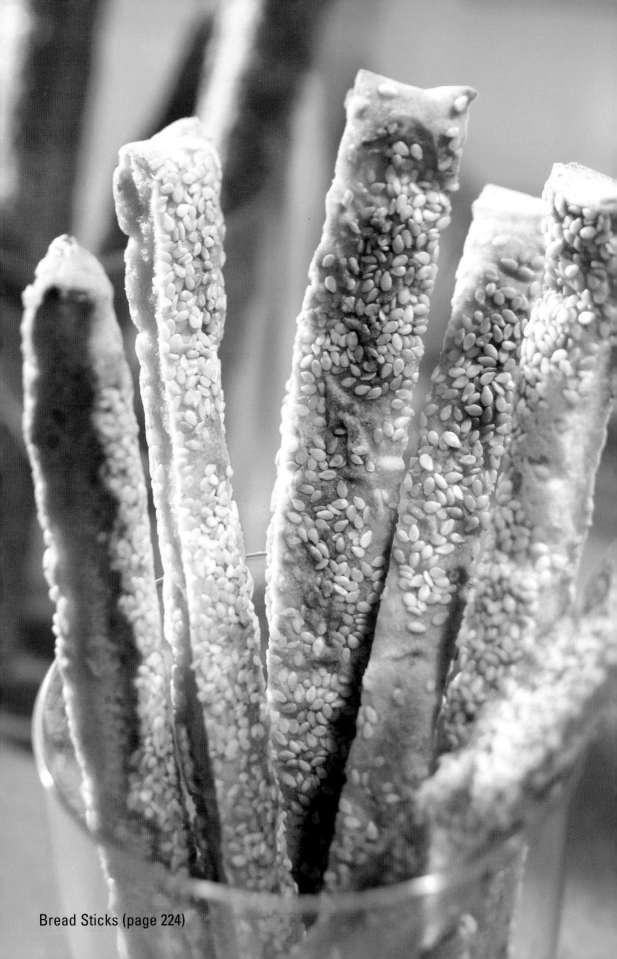

Bread Sticks (page 224)

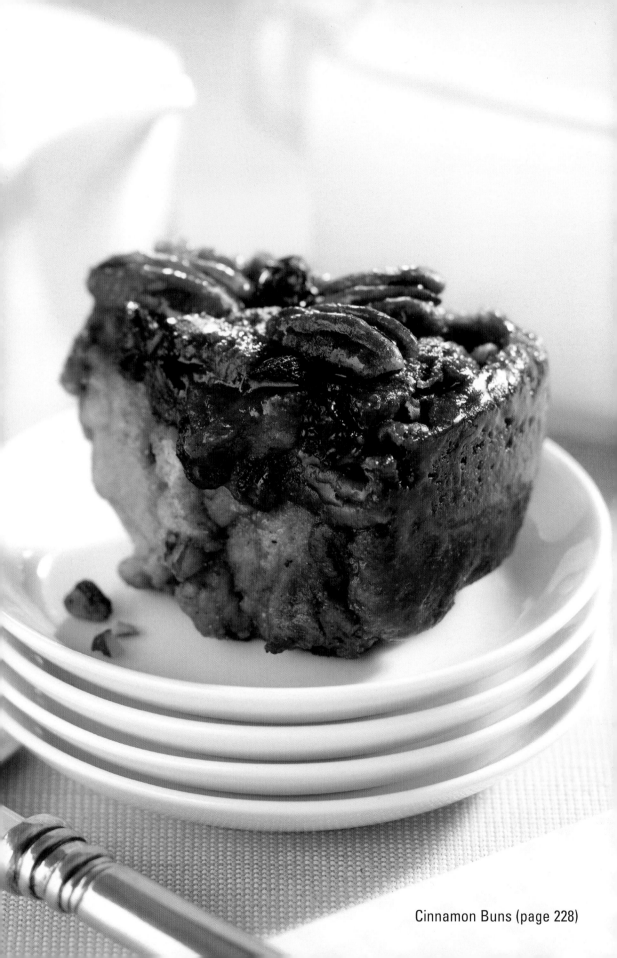

Cinnamon Buns (page 228)

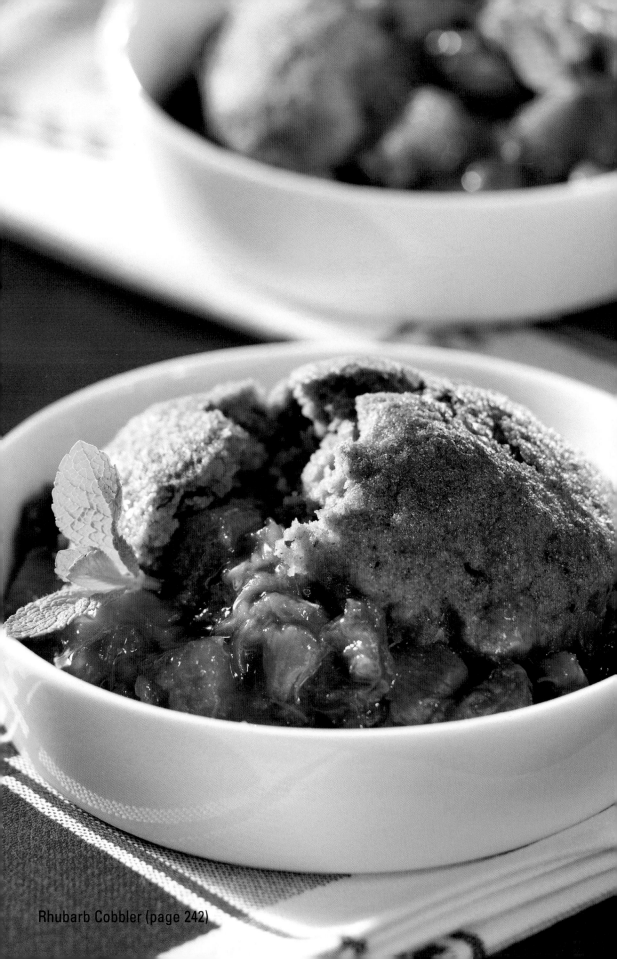

Rhubarb Cobbler (page 242)

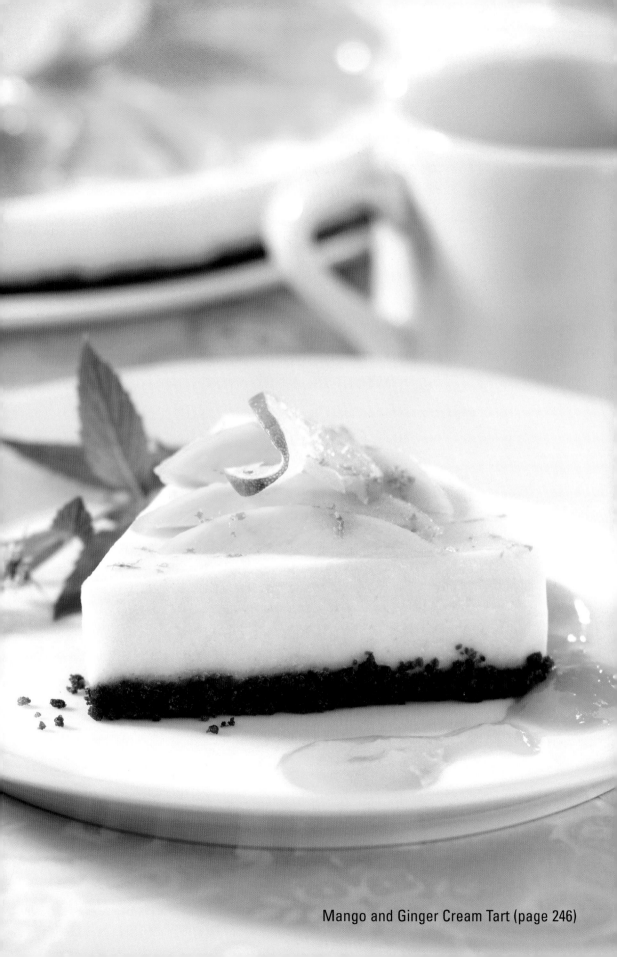

Mango and Ginger Cream Tart (page 246)

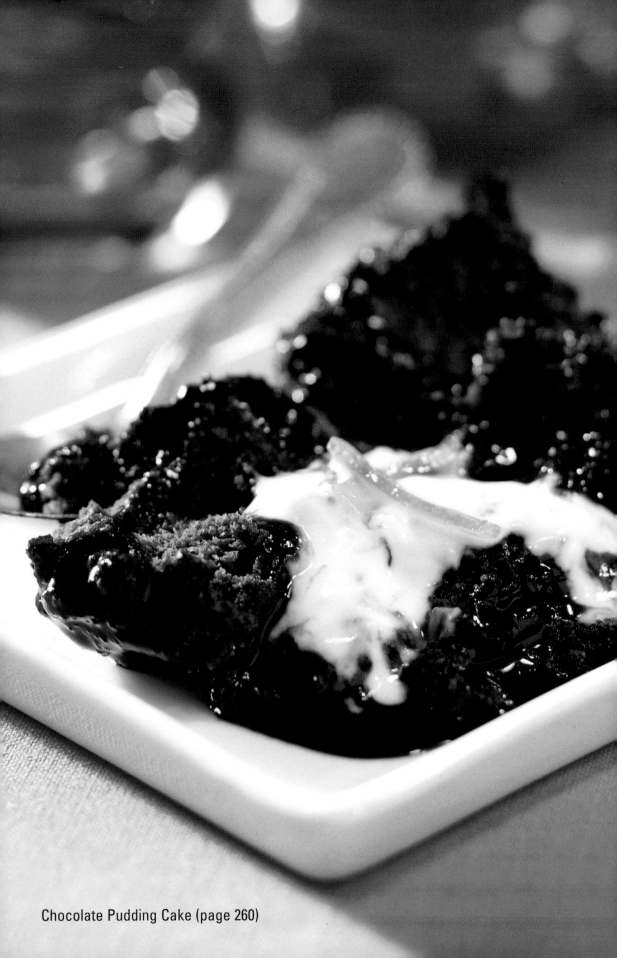

Chocolate Pudding Cake (page 260)

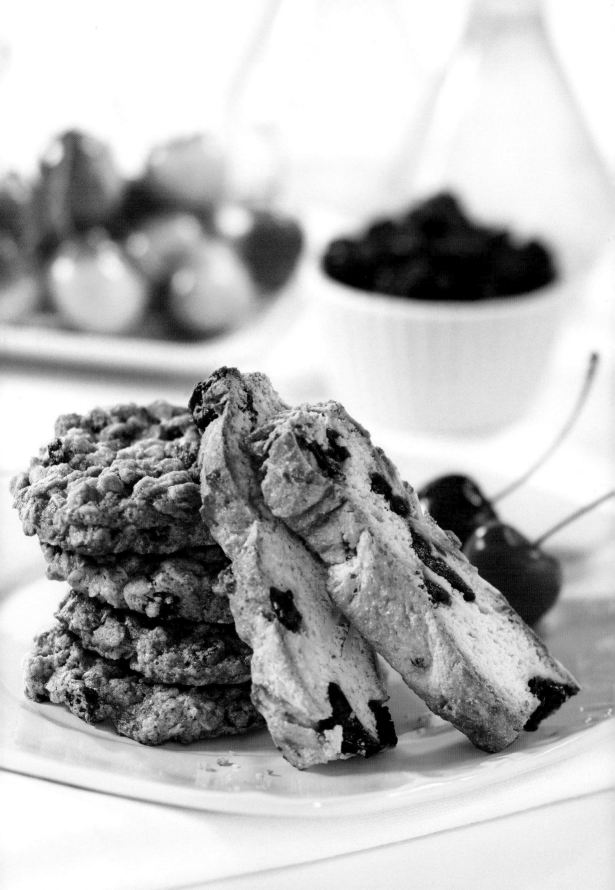

Oatmeal Raisin Cookies (page 268) and Cherry Almond Biscotti (page 274)

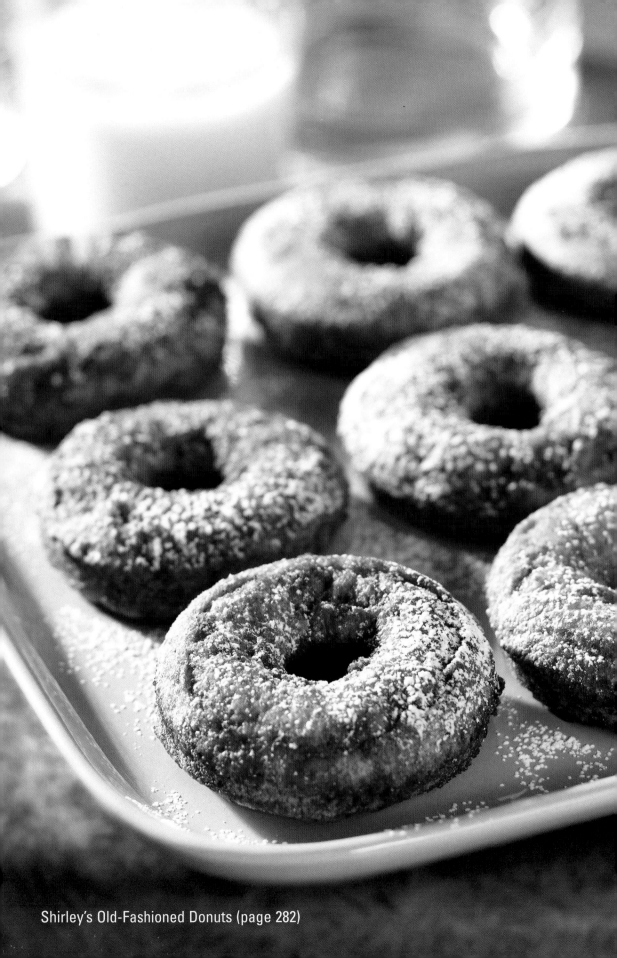

Shirley's Old-Fashioned Donuts (page 282)

Cherry Walnut Pie

Makes 10 servings

This recipe is the perfect filling for Chocolate Walnut Crust (page 237).

Tips

For easy serving, cut into wedges with a serrated knife dipped in hot water.

For information on toasting walnuts, see under Nuts in the Technique Glossary, page 301.

♦ *Preheat oven to 350°F (180°C)*

½ cup	packed brown sugar	125 mL
½ cup	corn syrup	125 mL
1 tbsp	buttery spread or butter, softened	15 mL
1 tbsp	cornstarch	15 mL
2	eggs	2
1 tsp	vanilla	5 mL
1½ cups	walnut pieces, toasted	375 mL
½ cup	chopped dried cherries	125 mL
1	Chocolate Walnut Crust, unbaked (see recipe, page 237)	1

1. In a large bowl, using an electric mixer, beat brown sugar, corn syrup, buttery spread and cornstarch until combined. Beat in eggs and vanilla. Stir in walnuts and cherries. Spoon into unbaked crust.

2. Bake in preheated oven for 40 to 45 minutes, or until filling is firm to the touch. (If crust is getting too dark, shield edges with strips of foil during the last 15 minutes of baking.) Filling may wobble in center but sets upon cooling. Refrigerate for about 4 hours, until set, or overnight.

Variation

Substitute dried cranberries for the cherries.

NUTRITIONAL VALUE
per serving

Calories	402
Fat, total	23 g
Fat, saturated	3 g
Cholesterol	37 mg
Sodium	134 mg
Carbohydrate	49 g
Fiber	3 g
Protein	7 g
Calcium	47 mg
Iron	2 mg

Rhubarb Cobbler

Makes 4 to 5 servings

Plan to serve this classic dessert on a chilly late spring day.

Tip

Be sure cobbler topping is ready to put on the hot rhubarb. If by chance the base cools, reheat until steaming. The bottom of the cobbler cooks from the heat of the rhubarb.

NUTRITIONAL VALUE per serving	
Calories	378
Fat, total	10 g
Fat, saturated	1 g
Cholesterol	37 mg
Sodium	140 mg
Carbohydrate	72 g
Fiber	5 g
Protein	4 g
Calcium	339 mg
Iron	2 mg

♦ Preheat oven to 400°F (200°C)
♦ 8-cup (2 L) straight-sided casserole, lightly greased

Base

5 cups	chopped fresh rhubarb	1.25 L
¾ cup	liquid honey	175 mL

Topping

½ cup	sorghum flour	125 mL
3 tbsp	quinoa flour	45 mL
2 tbsp	tapioca starch	50 mL
⅓ cup	packed brown sugar	75 mL
½ tsp	xanthan gum	2 mL
1 tsp	GF baking powder	5 mL
¼ tsp	salt	1 mL
½ tsp	ground cinnamon	2 mL
Pinch	ground cloves	Pinch
3 tbsp	vegetable oil	45 mL
⅓ cup	unsweetened applesauce	75 mL
½ tsp	vanilla	2 mL
1	egg	1

1. *Prepare the base:* In prepared casserole, toss together rhubarb and honey. Bake in preheated oven for 20 to 25 minutes, or until steaming. Reduce oven temperature to 350°F (180°C).

2. *Meanwhile, prepare the topping:* In a small bowl or plastic bag, combine sorghum flour, quinoa flour, tapioca starch, brown sugar, xanthan gum, baking powder, salt, cinnamon and cloves. Mix well and set aside.

3. In a large bowl, using an electric mixer, beat oil, applesauce, vanilla and egg until combined. Add dry ingredients and mix just until combined.

Be sure to use
unsweetened applesauce
in this recipe. If only
sweetened applesauce
is available, decrease the
brown sugar to $\frac{1}{4}$ cup
(50 mL).

4. Drop topping by heaping spoonfuls over hot rhubarb
   in pan, leaving it rough and rounded, with space
   between each spoonful.

5. Bake for 25 to 35 minutes, or until a tester inserted in
   the center comes out clean. Serve warm.

To make this recipe egg-free
Omit egg from recipe. Add 1 tsp (5 mL) powdered
egg replacer with the dry ingredients and add
2 tbsp (25 mL) water with the liquids.

Variation
Use frozen rhubarb, thawed and drained, instead of
fresh; decrease the honey to $\frac{1}{2}$ cup (125 mL).

Medley of Fruit Crisp

Makes 4 servings

Old-fashioned, but never out of fashion, this dessert is truly a comfort food!

Tips

If you are not familiar with cardamom, it has a strong, warmly spiced flavor that you may enjoy. It's often used in Scandinavian and Indian cuisines. Cinnamon, ginger or nutmeg can be used as a substitute.

If you use a smaller or deeper casserole dish, the baking time may be up to twice as long.

If you cannot tolerate cornstarch, substitute an equal amount of arrowroot starch.

> ♦ *Preheat oven to 375°F (190°C)*
> ♦ *8-cup (2 L) shallow casserole dish, lightly greased*

Base

4 cups	frozen unsweetened mixed peaches, blackberries and strawberries	1 L
2 tbsp	cornstarch	25 mL
2 tbsp	granulated sugar	25 mL

Topping

1½ cups	GF oats	375 mL
⅓ cup	GF oat flour	75 mL
3 tbsp	packed brown sugar	45 mL
1 tsp	ground cardamom	5 mL
⅓ cup	buttery spread or butter, melted	75 mL

1. *Prepare the base:* In prepared casserole dish, combine fruit, cornstarch and sugar. Bake in preheated oven for 30 minutes, or until fruit begins to thicken and steam.

2. *Meanwhile, prepare the topping:* In a medium bowl, combine oats, oat flour, brown sugar and cardamom. Drizzle with buttery spread and mix until crumbly. Sprinkle topping over hot fruit. Do not pack.

3. Bake for 25 to 30 minutes, or until fruit is bubbly around the edges, juices are thickened and clear, a tester inserted in the center is hot to the touch and topping is browned. Serve warm.

NUTRITIONAL VALUE
per serving

Calories	437
Fat, total	12 g
Fat, saturated	3 g
Cholesterol	0 mg
Sodium	88 mg
Carbohydrate	72 g
Fiber	11 g
Protein	8 g
Calcium	60 mg
Iron	5 mg

Variations

You can use other mixed fruit combinations; the baking time will vary according to the type of fruit selected. If using larger fruit pieces, increase the baking time.

Instead of baking, microwave base, uncovered, on High for 5 minutes. Stir and microwave on High for 5 minutes, or until fruit is steaming. Sprinkle topping over hot fruit. Microwave on High for 7 minutes. Let stand for 5 minutes.

Rum and Pecan Pie

Makes 6 to 8 servings

Enjoy pecan pie but sometimes find it too rich? Try our version. The rum smoothes the flavor and cuts the sweetness.

Tip

We have basic pie crust recipes in our earlier gluten-free cookbooks. The one in *125 Best Gluten-Free Recipes* uses rice flour with shortening; the one in *The Best Gluten-Free Family Cookbook* uses sorghum flour with vegetable oil. Both books have lots of extra tips and hints for making a pie crust. If you're short on time, or don't have either of these books, you can use a store-bought GF pie shell.

♦ *Preheat oven to 375°F (190°C)*

3	eggs	3
1 cup	packed brown sugar	250 mL
½ cup	dark corn syrup	125 mL
¼ tsp	salt	1 mL
2 tbsp	dark rum	25 mL
¼ cup	melted buttery spread or butter	50 mL
1	9-inch (23 cm) single-crust pie shell, unbaked (see tip, at left)	1
1 cup	pecan halves	250 mL

1. In a large bowl, using an electric mixer, beat eggs for 3 to 5 minutes, or until light lemon in color and fluffy. Stir in brown sugar, corn syrup, salt and rum until thoroughly combined. Stir in melted buttery spread. Pour into unbaked pie shell. Top with pecan halves.

2. Bake in preheated oven for 30 to 40 minutes, or until a knife inserted in the center comes out clean. Let cool completely on a rack.

Variation

Substitute orange juice for the rum.

Pecan Nutritional Value

Pecans contain more than 19 vitamins and minerals, including vitamins A and E, folate, calcium, magnesium, phosphorus, potassium, several B vitamins and zinc. Half the fat is monounsaturated and a quarter is polyunsaturated. Pecans contain antioxidants that may have a protective effect against certain cancers and heart disease and that aid in lowering cholesterol. Pecans are a source of protein and also increase fiber when added to breads and other baked goods.

NUTRITIONAL VALUE per serving	
Calories	416
Fat, total	20 g
Fat, saturated	4 g
Cholesterol	70 mg
Sodium	313 mg
Carbohydrate	55 g
Fiber	1 g
Protein	5 g
Calcium	47 mg
Iron	2 mg

Mango and Ginger Cream Tart

Makes 12 servings

Ginger and mangoes pair up perfectly in this delicious dessert.

Tips

To help filling cool quickly, saucepan can be set in a sink or a larger saucepan of cold water. Make sure the water level is about the same as the level of filling in the pan.

This is the perfect recipe in which to use Naturegg Break-Free liquid eggs; use ³⁄₄ cup (175 mL).

♦ *8-inch (20 cm) or 9-inch (23 cm) springform pan*

Crust

1¾ cups	Gingerbread Crumbs (see recipe, page 238)	425 mL
2 tbsp	buttery spread or butter, melted	25 mL

Ginger Cream

¼ cup	amaranth flour	50 mL
¾ cup	granulated sugar	175 mL
3 cups	fortified soy beverage, lactose-free milk or milk	750 mL
3	eggs, lightly beaten	3
1	envelope (¼ oz/7g) unflavored gelatin	1
3 tbsp	minced candied ginger	45 mL
1 tbsp	vanilla	15 mL
1	mango, sliced	1
	Mango Purée (see recipe, page 288)	

1. *Prepare the crust:* In a small bowl, combine gingerbread crumbs and buttery spread; mix well. Press crumbs into bottom of pan. Refrigerate until chilled, about 15 minutes.

2. *Prepare the ginger cream:* In a large heavy saucepan, stir together amaranth flour and sugar; gradually stir in soy beverage and eggs. Sprinkle with unflavored gelatin and let stand for 10 minutes. Cook over medium heat, stirring constantly, for about 15 minutes, or until just thick enough to coat a metal spoon. Do not let boil. Remove from heat and stir in ginger and vanilla. Place saucepan in cold water (see tip, at left) and stir until ginger cream no longer steams.

3. Spoon ginger cream into chilled crust, smoothing top. Cover and refrigerate for at least 3 hours, until set, or overnight.

NUTRITIONAL VALUE
per serving

Calories	230
Fat, total	7 g
Fat, saturated	2 g
Cholesterol	48 mg
Sodium	118 mg
Carbohydrate	37 g
Fiber	1 g
Protein	5 g
Calcium	113 mg
Iron	2 mg

This dessert (un-garnished) can be wrapped airtight and frozen for up to 1 month. To serve, let stand at room temperature for at least 30 minutes before slicing. Slice with a sharp knife dipped in hot water. Garnish with mango slices and Mango Purée just before serving.

4. Cover filling with overlapping mango slices. Drizzle individual servings with Mango Purée.

Variation

Substitute 4 large fresh peaches for the mango in the tart, and use the peach variation of the Mango Purée recipe (page 288) for the purée.

Mangoes

Mangoes can be as small as an egg or as heavy as 5 pounds (2.3 kg), and can be oval, round or kidney-shaped. They have a large, tongue-shaped pit surrounded by flesh that ranges in color from yellow to red. Mangoes are picked unripe and should be firm, with green skin and no blemishes. When ripe, they are completely colored with areas of green, yellow and red and should be quite firm to the touch, with a sweet, fruity smell.

Ripen mangoes in a paper bag at room temperature for 3 to 5 days. Once ripe, they can be refrigerated in a plastic bag for up to 1 week.

Flavors that combine well with mangoes are apricot, avocado, bell pepper, chicken, chili pepper, cilantro, cucumber, fish, lime juice, orange, passion fruit, pineapple, rum, seafood and star fruit.

To pit and slice a mango, lay it narrow side up on a cutting board. Cut flesh from each side of the pit and discard pit, then slice flesh lengthwise. To cube, after pitting, cut a grid pattern in the flesh, down to (but not through) the skin. Gently push skin to turn inside out; cut off flesh.

You can also try using a mango splitter, a tool similar in appearance to an apple corer. Its sharp, elliptical, centered metal blade slides down around the pit, slicing the fruit in half at the same time. Two handles, opposite each other, prevent your hands from slipping. It works best on large mangoes.

Pear Hazelnut Tart

Makes 12 servings

Enjoy this elegant, soft-textured fruity tart in a not-too-crisp hazelnut crumb crust — we've adapted it from a recipe in *Homemakers* magazine to make it gluten-free and lactose-free, just for you.

Tips

For instructions on toasting hazelnut flour, see the Technique Glossary, page 300.

Use a small spoon or melon baller to scoop out the core of the pears.

To space pear halves evenly, imagine a clock. Place pear halves at 12, 3, 6 and 9, then place remaining pear halves in between.

NUTRITIONAL VALUE per serving	
Calories	226
Fat, total	12 g
Fat, saturated	1 g
Cholesterol	0 mg
Sodium	133 mg
Carbohydrate	27 g
Fiber	3 g
Protein	4 g
Calcium	47 mg
Iron	4 mg

◆ *Preheat oven to 350°F (180°C)*
◆ *9-inch (23 cm) springform pan*
◆ *Rimmed baking sheet*

Crust

2 cups	hazelnut flour, toasted	500 mL
¾ tsp	ground cardamom	4 mL
¼ cup	liquid honey	50 mL

Filling

4	firm Bosc pears	4
⅔ cup	lactose-free plain yogurt or plain yogurt	150 mL
⅔ cup	fortified soy beverage, lactose-free milk or milk	150 mL
1	package (3 oz/102 g) GF vanilla instant pudding mix	1
2 tbsp	hazelnut-flavored liqueur, such as Frangelico	25 mL

1. Cut a 15-inch (38 cm) length of parchment paper. Center over the bottom plate of springform pan and close hinge of rim to hold paper in place. Trim off excess parchment paper.

2. *Prepare the crust:* In a medium bowl, combine hazelnut flour, cardamom and honey; mix well. Press crumbs into bottom of prepared pan. Bake in preheated oven for 8 to 10 minutes, or until lightly browned. Let cool. Preheat broiler.

3. *Prepare the filling:* Peel pears, halve lengthwise, scoop out the core and remove stem. Place one half on cutting board, cut side down. Using a sharp knife, slice thinly, crosswise, keeping shape intact. Gently press down on sliced pear half, fanning the slices toward the wide end. Slide a metal spatula under pear half and transfer to rimmed baking sheet. Repeat with remaining pear halves.

4. Broil pears for 8 to 10 minutes, or until golden brown on top and tender. Let cool on baking sheet.

Tips

When transferring pear halves from baking sheet to tart, use a knife to gently push the pear off the spatula onto the pudding mixture.

If you don't have a metal spatula, use a palette knife, a French knife, a Santoku knife or a pie server to lift the pears.

5. In a medium bowl, using an electric mixer on low speed, beat yogurt, soy beverage, pudding mix and liqueur for about 2 minutes, or until smooth. Spread over cooled crust. Refrigerate until chilled, about 10 minutes.

6. Slide metal spatula under one pear half and transfer to tart, with the narrow end facing the center. Repeat with remaining pear halves, spacing evenly. Refrigerate for 30 minutes, until filling is set, or for up to 24 hours.

Variation

Substitute apple, orange or pear juice for the Frangelico.

Linzertorte

Makes 9 to 12 servings

We modified Martha Stewart's recipe to make it gluten-free just for you! We even made an egg-free version. A traditional Viennese linzertorte is round, but you can bake it in a 9-inch (23 cm) square pan if you like.

Tips

For instructions on toasting almond flour, see the Technique Glossary, page 299.

Use a raspberry jam with a thick consistency. We tried several types of jam and preferred an extra fruit, sugar-reduced one.

NUTRITIONAL VALUE per serving

Calories	262
Fat, total	7 g
Fat, saturated	1 g
Cholesterol	16 mg
Sodium	152 mg
Carbohydrate	47 g
Fiber	1 g
Protein	4 g
Calcium	58 mg
Iron	1 mg

♦ 9-inch (23 cm) round silicone baking pan with 2-inch (5 cm) sides, or 9-inch (23 cm) springform pan

1 cup	almond flour, toasted	250 mL
¾ cup	brown rice flour	175 mL
¼ cup	soy flour	50 mL
¼ cup	tapioca starch	50 mL
1 tsp	xanthan gum	5 mL
½ tsp	GF baking powder	2 mL
½ tsp	salt	2 mL
¼ tsp	ground cinnamon	1 mL
Pinch	ground cloves	Pinch
⅓ cup	buttery spread or butter, softened	75 mL
⅔ cup	packed brown sugar	150 mL
1 tsp	grated lemon zest	5 mL
1	egg	1
1¼ cups	raspberry jam	300 mL
	GF confectioner's (icing) sugar, sifted	

1. In a medium bowl or plastic bag, combine almond flour, brown rice flour, soy flour, tapioca starch, xanthan gum, baking powder, salt, cinnamon and cloves. Mix well and set aside.

2. In a large bowl, using an electric mixer, cream buttery spread, brown sugar and lemon zest. Add egg; cream until light and fluffy. Add dry ingredients and mix on low just until mixture comes together to form a dough.

3. Divide dough into thirds. Place each ball on plastic wrap, flatten into a disk ⅛ inch (3 mm) thick and wrap airtight. Refrigerate for at least 30 minutes, until chilled, or overnight. Preheat oven to 350°F (180°C).

4. Press 2 of the 3 disks into the bottom and 1 inch (2.5 cm) up the sides of the pan to form a shell. Spread jam evenly over the bottom of the shell.

5. Using a pastry cutter or pizza wheel, cut the remaining chilled disk into ½-inch (1 cm) wide strips. Arrange pastry strips over top of jam in a lattice pattern.

If you prefer a seedless jam, place jam in a saucepan over low heat to melt, then strain through a fine sieve. Let cool slightly before spreading. (Or look for seedless raspberry jam.)

6. Bake for 35 to 45 minutes, or until pastry is golden brown and jam is bubbling. Let cool completely in pan on a rack. Just before serving, lightly dust with confectioner's sugar.

To make this recipe egg-free
Omit egg from recipe. Combine 2 tbsp (25 mL) flax flour or ground flaxseed with 3 tbsp (45 mL) warm water. Let stand for 5 minutes. Add to brown sugar mixture.

Variations

Apricot, blueberry, mixed berry or bumbleberry jam can be substituted for the raspberry jam.

Substitute hazelnut or pecan flour for the almond flour.

Banana Cake with Coconut Topping

Makes 12 to 16 servings

More like banana bread than banana cake, this snacking cake brings back fond memories of the Hawaiian Islands for us.

Tip

Bake in center of oven — we found that the bottom browned a lot quicker when we used a modern thin cake pan than with an old heavier one.

◆ *9-inch (2.5 L) square baking pan, lightly greased*

Cake

1 cup	sorghum flour	250 mL
1/3 cup	soy flour	75 mL
2 tbsp	tapioca starch	25 mL
1 1/2 tsp	xanthan gum	7 mL
1 tbsp	GF baking powder	15 mL
1/4 tsp	salt	1 mL
1/4 cup	soy milk powder or nonfat (skim) milk powder	50 mL
1/4 cup	vegetable oil	50 mL
1/4 cup	water	50 mL
1 1/4 cups	mashed bananas	300 mL
1/2 cup	granulated sugar	125 mL
1 tsp	vanilla	5 mL
2	eggs	2

Topping

3/4 cup	shredded unsweetened coconut	175 mL
1/4 cup	packed brown sugar	50 mL
1/2 tsp	ground nutmeg	2 mL
2 tbsp	lactose-free margarine or margarine, melted	25 mL

1. *Prepare the cake:* In a medium bowl or plastic bag, combine sorghum flour, soy flour, tapioca starch, xanthan gum, baking powder, salt and soy milk powder. Mix well and set aside.

2. In a large bowl, using an electric mixer, beat oil, water, bananas, sugar, vanilla and eggs until combined. Add dry ingredients and mix just until combined.

3. Spoon batter into prepared pan. Using a moistened rubber spatula, spread to edges and smooth top.

NUTRITIONAL VALUE per serving

Calories	196
Fat, total	7 g
Fat, saturated	2 g
Cholesterol	23 mg
Sodium	62 mg
Carbohydrate	27 g
Fiber	2 g
Protein	8 g
Calcium	81 mg
Iron	2 mg

Tip

If coconut topping is toasting and browning quickly after 20 minutes, tent cake with foil.

4. *Prepare the topping:* In a small bowl, stir together coconut, brown sugar and nutmeg. Drizzle with melted margarine and mix until crumbly. Sprinkle over batter. Let stand for 30 minutes. Meanwhile, preheat oven to 350°F (180°C).

5. Bake for 35 to 45 minutes, or until a tester inserted in the center comes out clean. Let cool completely in pan on a rack.

To make this recipe egg-free
Omit eggs from recipe. Add 2 tsp (10 mL) powdered egg replacer with the dry ingredients and increase water to $\frac{1}{2}$ cup (125 mL).

Variations

To make a spicier version, add 1 tsp (5 mL) ground cinnamon, an extra $\frac{1}{4}$ tsp (1 mL) ground nutmeg and a pinch of ground allspice.

For a higher cake, bake in an 8-inch (2 L) square baking pan for 45 to 55 minutes.

Lemon Cheesecake

Makes 4 servings

We thought long and hard about what flavor of cheesecake to include in this book. We've settled on lemon — enjoy! Serve with raspberries, blueberries, chocolate sauce or our Lotsa Lemon Sauce (page 130 of *125 Best Gluten-Free Recipes*).

Tips

Drain the tofu well in a sieve; otherwise, the cheesecake may not set properly. For more information on tofu, see pages 52–53.

After you turn the oven off, be sure to set a kitchen timer for the time the cheesecake needs to cool in the oven. It's easy to forget all about it!

* Preheat oven to 325°F (160°C)
* 5½-inch (15 cm) springform pan, lightly greased

Crust

½ cup	Gingerbread Crumbs (see recipe, page 238)	125 mL
1 tbsp	buttery spread or butter, melted	15 mL

Filling

1	package (12 oz/340 g) firm silken tofu, well drained	1
2	eggs	2
½ cup	granulated sugar	125 mL
1 tbsp	grated lemon zest	15 mL
1 tbsp	freshly squeezed lemon juice	15 mL
2 tbsp	amaranth flour	25 mL

1. *Prepare the crust:* In a small bowl, combine Gingerbread Crumbs and buttery spread; mix well. Press crumbs into bottom of prepared pan. Refrigerate until chilled, about 15 minutes.

2. *Prepare the filling:* In a food processor fitted with a metal blade, purée tofu, scraping down sides frequently, for 1 to 3 minutes, or until smooth. Add eggs, sugar, lemon zest, lemon juice and amaranth flour; process until smooth.

3. Spoon filling into chilled crust, smoothing top.

4. Bake in preheated oven for 40 to 45 minutes, or until all but the center 1 inch (2.5 cm) is set. Turn the oven off, but leave cheesecake in for 30 minutes (this helps prevent large cracks). Let cool completely in pan on a rack, then remove ring of pan. Refrigerate for at least 4 hours or overnight.

NUTRITIONAL VALUE
per serving

Calories	298
Fat, total	11 g
Fat, saturated	3 g
Cholesterol	94 mg
Sodium	130 mg
Carbohydrate	41 g
Fiber	1 g
Protein	10 g
Calcium	62 mg
Iron	3 mg

Tip

Recipe can be doubled and baked in a 9-inch (23 cm) springform pan. Increase the baking time by 5 to 10 minutes.

Variations

Substitute GF white cake crumbs for the Gingerbread Crumbs (see page 142 in *125 Best Gluten-Free Recipes* for a white cake recipe).

If you prefer, you can prepare this cheesecake in a 9- by 5-inch (2 L) loaf pan. Decrease the baking time by about 5 minutes.

If you can tolerate lactose, substitute two 8-oz (250 g) packages of cream cheese, softened, for the silken tofu. Do not substitute with lactose-free cream cheese — when heated, it has a tendency to curdle.

Lemon Hazelnut Coffee Cake

Makes 9 to 12 servings

The combination of hazelnuts and lemon is always a hit. We like to serve this cake warm. It also makes a great snack to carry when traveling.

Tips

For information on making your own hazelnut flour, see under Nut flour in the Technique Glossary, page 301.

One lemon yields about 1 tbsp (15 mL) of zest. It's worth the time and effort it takes to zest fresh lemons and squeeze the fresh juice. Freeze any extra zest and juice for next time.

Use a sharp knife rather than a food processor to chop the hazelnuts.

NUTRITIONAL VALUE per serving

Calories	313
Fat, total	16 g
Fat, saturated	1 g
Cholesterol	16 mg
Sodium	114 mg
Carbohydrate	41 g
Fiber	3 g
Protein	6 g
Calcium	111 mg
Iron	2 mg

♦ 9-inch (2.5 L) square baking pan, lightly greased

1½ cups	sorghum flour	375 mL
⅔ cup	hazelnut flour	150 mL
½ cup	tapioca starch	125 mL
1½ tsp	xanthan gum	7 mL
1 tbsp	GF baking powder	15 mL
½ tsp	salt	2 mL
1 cup	fortified soy beverage, lactose-free milk or milk	250 mL
1 cup	granulated sugar	250 mL
¼ cup	vegetable oil	50 mL
1 tbsp	vanilla	15 mL
⅓ cup	grated lemon zest	75 mL
¼ cup	freshly squeezed lemon juice	50 mL
1	egg	1
1 cup	chopped hazelnuts	250 mL

1. In a medium bowl or plastic bag, combine sorghum flour, hazelnut flour, tapioca starch, xanthan gum, baking powder and salt. Mix well and set aside.

2. In a large bowl, using an electric mixer, beat soy beverage, sugar, oil, vanilla, lemon zest, lemon juice and egg until combined. Add dry ingredients and mix just until combined. Stir in hazelnuts.

3. Spoon batter into prepared pan. Using a moistened rubber spatula, spread to edges and smooth top. Let stand for 30 minutes. Meanwhile, preheat oven to 350°F (180°C).

4. Bake for 45 to 55 minutes, or until a tester inserted in the center comes out clean. Let cool in pan on a rack for 10 minutes. Serve warm.

> **To make this recipe egg-free**
> Omit egg from recipe. Combine ¼ cup (50 mL) flax flour or ground flaxseed with ⅓ cup (75 mL) warm water. Let stand for 5 minutes. Add with vanilla.

Chocolate Ginger Cake

Makes 12 servings

Friends and family will never guess the secret to this egg-free cake's moistness: apple juice! It's low in fat and high in flavor — and gluten-free, to boot.

Tip

When using a dark-colored springform pan, decrease the oven temperature by 25°F (14°C). We do this with our glass-bottomed pans as well.

♦ 9-inch (23 cm) springform pan, lightly greased

Cake

¾ cup	sorghum flour	175 mL
⅔ cup	whole bean flour	150 mL
⅓ cup	potato starch	75 mL
⅔ cup	packed brown sugar	150 mL
1½ tsp	xanthan gum	7 mL
2 tsp	GF baking powder	10 mL
½ tsp	baking soda	2 mL
¼ tsp	salt	1 mL
¼ cup	unsweetened cocoa powder, sifted	50 mL
1 tbsp	ground ginger	15 mL
¾ tsp	ground cinnamon	4 mL
1 cup	unsweetened apple juice	250 mL
3 tbsp	vegetable oil	45 mL

Topping

½ cup	chopped crystallized ginger	125 mL
1 cup	pecan pieces	250 mL
¼ cup	packed brown sugar	50 mL
¼ tsp	ground cinnamon	1 mL

1. *Prepare the cake:* In a large bowl or plastic bag, combine sorghum flour, whole bean flour, potato starch, brown sugar, xanthan gum, baking powder, baking soda, salt, cocoa, ginger and cinnamon. Mix well and set aside.

2. In a separate bowl, using an electric mixer, beat apple juice and oil until combined. Add dry ingredients and mix just until combined.

3. Spoon batter into prepared pan. Using a moistened rubber spatula, spread to edges and smooth top. Let stand for 30 minutes. Meanwhile, preheat oven to 350°F (180°C).

4. *Prepare the topping:* In a small bowl, stir together ginger, pecans, brown sugar and cinnamon. Sprinkle topping over batter. Do not pack.

5. Bake for 35 to 40 minutes, or until a tester inserted in the center comes out clean. Let cool completely in pan on a rack.

NUTRITIONAL VALUE
per serving

Calories	233
Fat, total	10 g
Fat, saturated	1 g
Cholesterol	0 mg
Sodium	112 mg
Carbohydrate	36 g
Fiber	2 g
Protein	3 g
Calcium	70 mg
Iron	2 mg

Chocolate Banana Snacking Cake

Makes 9 to 12 servings

There's no need to ice this moist cake with a strong banana flavor. It's perfect for packed lunches or after-school snacks.

Tip

For instructions on mashing and freezing overripe bananas, see the Technique Glossary, page 299.

♦ 8-inch (2 L) square baking pan, lightly greased and bottom lined with parchment paper

⅔ cup	sorghum flour	150 mL
¼ cup	quinoa flour	50 mL
2 tbsp	tapioca starch	25 mL
1½ tsp	xanthan gum	7 mL
2 tsp	GF baking powder	10 mL
½ tsp	baking soda	2 mL
¼ tsp	salt	1 mL
⅓ cup	unsweetened cocoa powder, sifted	75 mL
1 cup	mashed bananas	250 mL
¾ cup	granulated sugar	175 mL
⅓ cup	vegetable oil	75 mL
¼ cup	water	50 mL
1 tsp	vanilla	5 mL
1	egg	1

1. In a medium bowl or plastic bag, combine sorghum flour, quinoa flour, tapioca starch, xanthan gum, baking powder, baking soda, salt and cocoa. Mix well and set aside.

2. In a large bowl, using an electric mixer, beat bananas, sugar, oil, water, vanilla and egg until combined. Add dry ingredients and mix just until combined.

3. Spoon batter into prepared pan. Using a moistened rubber spatula, spread to edges and smooth top. Let stand for 30 minutes. Meanwhile, preheat oven to 350°F (180°C).

4. Bake for 35 to 45 minutes, or until a tester inserted in the center comes out clean. Let cool in pan on a rack for 10 minutes. Remove from pan and let cool completely on rack.

NUTRITIONAL VALUE per serving	
Calories	175
Fat, total	7 g
Fat, saturated	1 g
Cholesterol	16 mg
Sodium	109 mg
Carbohydrate	28 g
Fiber	2 g
Protein	2 g
Calcium	46 mg
Iron	1 mg

To make this recipe egg-free

Omit egg from recipe. Add 1 tsp (5 mL) powdered egg replacer with the dry ingredients and increase the water to $\frac{1}{3}$ cup (75 mL).

Variations

For a stronger chocolate and milder banana flavor, increase the cocoa powder to $\frac{1}{2}$ cup (125 mL).

If quinoa flour is not available, substitute an equal amount of brown rice flour.

Chocolate Pudding Cake

<table>
<tr><td>

Makes 4 to 6 servings

</td></tr>
</table>

A comforting finale to the coldest winter day, this old-fashioned, self-saucing dessert was all the rage in the '50s. We've updated it and made it lactose-free and gluten-free.

Tip

When boiling the water, heat extra and measure after it has come to a boil. It may continue to bubble when removed from the stovetop or microwave, so be careful not to burn yourself.

♦ *Preheat oven to 350°F (180°C)*
♦ *6-cup (1.5 L) straight-sided casserole, lightly greased*

Cake

½ cup	sorghum flour	125 mL
¼ cup	whole bean flour	50 mL
½ cup	granulated sugar	125 mL
½ tsp	xanthan gum	2 mL
2 tsp	GF baking powder	10 mL
¼ cup	unsweetened cocoa powder, sifted	50 mL
1 cup	unsweetened applesauce	250 mL
2 tbsp	vegetable oil	25 mL
1 tsp	almond extract or vanilla	5 mL

Chocolate Sauce

¾ cup	packed brown sugar	175 mL
¼ cup	unsweetened cocoa powder, sifted	50 mL
1 cup	boiling water	250 mL

1. *Prepare the cake:* In a medium bowl or plastic bag, combine sorghum flour, whole bean flour, sugar, xanthan gum, baking powder and cocoa. Mix well and set aside.

2. In a large bowl, using an electric mixer, beat applesauce, oil and almond extract until combined. Slowly add dry ingredients and mix just until combined.

3. Spoon batter into prepared casserole.

4. *Prepare the chocolate sauce:* In a small bowl, combine brown sugar and cocoa. Sprinkle evenly over batter. Slowly pour boiling water evenly over batter. Do not stir.

5. Bake in preheated oven for 40 to 50 minutes, or until cake is firm when gently touched. Serve warm.

NUTRITIONAL VALUE
per serving

Calories	296
Fat, total	6 g
Fat, saturated	1 g
Cholesterol	0 mg
Sodium	16 mg
Carbohydrate	63 g
Fiber	4 g
Protein	3 g
Calcium	114 mg
Iron	2 mg

Makes 1$\frac{1}{2}$ cups (375 mL) ($\frac{1}{4}$ cup/50 mL per serving)

Caramel lovers can substitute this sauce for the chocolate sauce in Chocolate Pudding Cake (opposite).

Caramel Sauce

$\frac{3}{4}$ cup	packed brown sugar	175 mL
1 tbsp	lactose-free buttery spread or butter	15 mL
1 cup	boiling water	250 mL

1. Combine brown sugar, buttery spread and boiling water. Pour evenly over chocolate cake batter. Do not stir. Immediately bake in preheated oven for 40 to 50 minutes, or until cake is firm when gently touched. Serve warm.

NUTRITIONAL VALUE per serving

Calories	120
Fat, total	2 g
Fat, saturated	1 g
Cholesterol	0 mg
Sodium	32 mg
Carbohydrate	27 g
Fiber	0 g
Protein	0 g
Calcium	24 mg
Iron	1 mg

Cranberry Cake with Orange Sauce

Makes 9 servings

There's nothing better than the combination of cranberry and orange!

Tips

Cut large cranberries in half. They're easier to cut when frozen.

To partially thaw frozen cranberries, place in a single layer on a microwave-safe plate. Microwave on High for 1 minute, stirring once.

- 8-inch (2 L) square baking pan, lightly greased and lined with parchment paper

1¼ cups	sorghum flour	300 mL
¼ cup	quinoa flour	50 mL
¼ cup	tapioca starch	50 mL
1½ tsp	xanthan gum	7 mL
1 tbsp	GF baking powder	15 mL
½ tsp	salt	2 mL
1 tsp	ground cardamom or cinnamon	5 mL
¼ cup	vegetable oil	50 mL
⅔ cup	packed brown sugar	150 mL
1 tbsp	orange zest	15 mL
1 cup	freshly squeezed orange juice	250 mL
1 tsp	vanilla	5 mL
2 cups	fresh or frozen cranberries, partially thawed	500 mL
1	batch warm Orange Sauce (see recipe, opposite)	1

1. In a medium bowl or plastic bag, combine sorghum flour, quinoa flour, tapioca starch, xanthan gum, baking powder, salt and cardamom. Mix well and set aside.

2. In a large bowl, using an electric mixer, beat oil, brown sugar, orange zest, orange juice and vanilla until combined. Add dry ingredients and mix just until combined. Stir in cranberries.

3. Spoon batter into prepared pan. Using a moistened rubber spatula, spread to edges and smooth top. Let stand for 30 minutes. Meanwhile, preheat oven to 350°F (180°C).

4. Bake for 40 to 45 minutes, or until a tester inserted in the center comes out clean. Let cool in pan on a rack for 10 minutes. Remove from pan and let cool completely on rack. Serve each slice drizzled with 3 tbsp (45 mL) Orange Sauce.

NUTRITIONAL VALUE
per serving

Calories	240
Fat, total	7 g
Fat, saturated	0 g
Cholesterol	0 mg
Sodium	139 mg
Carbohydrate	44 g
Fiber	3 g
Protein	3 g
Calcium	101 mg
Iron	2 mg

Not too tangy, not too sweet, this refreshing citrus sauce pairs nicely with Cranberry Cake (opposite), as well as with Lemon Hazelnut Coffee Cake (page 256).

Tip

The flavor will vary depending on the type of orange juice used. We prefer to use freshly squeezed juice. You could try frozen reconstituted juice or juice from a carton, but avoid orange drink, as it is too sweet.

Orange Sauce

¾ cup	granulated sugar	175 mL
3 tbsp	cornstarch	45 mL
1 tbsp	grated orange zest	15 mL
1 cup	freshly squeezed orange juice	250 mL
1 cup	water	250 mL
2 tsp	lactose-free buttery spread or butter	10 mL

1. In a small saucepan, combine sugar, cornstarch and orange zest. Stir in orange juice and water. Bring to a boil over high heat, stirring constantly. Reduce heat to medium and simmer, stirring, for 2 to 3 minutes, or until slightly thickened and glossy. Remove from heat. Stir in buttery spread until it melts. Serve warm.

Variation

Add 2 tbsp (25 mL) orange-flavored liqueur such as Cointreau or Triple Sec with the buttery spread.

**NUTRITIONAL VALUE
per serving**

Calories	95
Fat, total	1 g
Fat, saturated	0 g
Cholesterol	0 mg
Sodium	10 mg
Carbohydrate	22 g
Fiber	0 g
Protein	0 g
Calcium	5 mg
Iron	0 mg

Date Orange Streusel Cake

Makes 12 servings

This moist cake is perfect to carry to a family get-together or celiac meeting.

Tip

If you can't tolerate oats, substitute buckwheat, amaranth or quinoa flakes for the GF oats. Stir in flakes after topping is crumbly, as they are more fragile than oats.

♦ 9-inch (2.5 L) square baking pan, lightly greased

Cake

1 cup	fortified soy beverage, lactose-free milk or milk	250 mL
1 tbsp	cider vinegar	15 mL
¾ cup	sorghum flour	175 mL
⅔ cup	whole bean flour	150 mL
¼ cup	tapioca starch	50 mL
1½ tsp	xanthan gum	7 mL
1 tbsp	GF baking powder	15 mL
1 tsp	baking soda	5 mL
½ tsp	salt	2 mL
½ tsp	ground cinnamon	2 mL
¼ tsp	ground ginger	1 mL
¼ tsp	ground nutmeg	1 mL
⅓ cup	vegetable oil	75 mL
⅔ cup	packed brown sugar	150 mL
2	eggs	2
2 tbsp	grated orange zest	25 mL
1 tsp	vanilla	5 mL
1½ cups	chopped dates	375 mL

Streusel Topping

⅔ cup	GF oats	150 mL
¼ cup	sorghum flour	50 mL
2 tbsp	buttery spread or butter, softened	25 mL
2 tbsp	packed brown sugar	25 mL
⅓ cup	pecan pieces	75 mL

1. *Prepare the cake:* In a measuring cup or bowl, combine soy beverage and vinegar. Set aside for 5 minutes.

2. In a large bowl or plastic bag, combine sorghum flour, whole bean flour, tapioca starch, xanthan gum, baking powder, baking soda, salt, cinnamon, ginger and nutmeg. Mix well and set aside.

NUTRITIONAL VALUE per serving

Calories	314
Fat, total	12 g
Fat, saturated	2 g
Cholesterol	31 mg
Sodium	250 mg
Carbohydrate	51 g
Fiber	4 g
Protein	5 g
Calcium	118 mg
Iron	2 mg

We use kitchen shears to snip whole dates into eighths, dipping shears in hot water as they become sticky. If you purchase chopped dates, check for wheat starch in the coating.

3. In a separate bowl, using an electric mixer, beat soy beverage mixture, oil, brown sugar, eggs, orange zest and vanilla until combined. Add dry ingredients and mix just until combined. Stir in dates.

4. Spoon batter into prepared pan. Spread to edges and smooth top.

5. *Prepare the streusel topping:* In a food processor fitted with a metal blade, pulse oats, sorghum flour, buttery spread, brown sugar and pecans 5 to 7 times, or just until crumbly. Don't over-pulse.

6. Sprinkle topping over batter and press slightly into batter. Let stand for 30 minutes. Meanwhile, preheat oven to 350°F (180°C).

7. Bake for 50 to 55 minutes, or until a tester inserted in the center comes out clean. Let cool completely in pan on a rack.

To make this recipe egg-free
Omit eggs from recipe. Combine $1/4$ cup (50 mL) flax flour or ground flaxseed with $1/2$ cup (125 mL) warm water. Let stand for 5 minutes. Add with vanilla.

Variation
Substitute $1\frac{1}{2}$ cups (375 mL) chopped dried figs for the dates.

Pineapple Yogurt Cupcakes

**Makes
12 cupcakes
(1 per serving)**

Looking for a light, moist, flavorful white cupcake to serve with seasonal fresh fruit? You've found it.

Tips

Fill each cup of the muffin tin almost level with the top.

Freeze these cupcakes individually for up to 1 month and include one for dessert in your lunch.

◆ *12-cup muffin tin, lightly greased*

⅔ cup	sorghum flour	150 mL
½ cup	amaranth flour	125 mL
⅓ cup	brown rice flour	75 mL
⅓ cup	tapioca starch	75 mL
¼ cup	granulated sugar	50 mL
1 tsp	xanthan gum	5 mL
2 tsp	GF baking powder	10 mL
1 tsp	baking soda	5 mL
½ tsp	salt	2 mL
½ tsp	ground nutmeg	2 mL
1	egg	1
1	egg white	1
¾ cup	crushed pineapple, including juice	175 mL
¼ cup	vegetable oil	50 mL
1 tsp	vanilla	5 mL
¾ cup	lactose-free plain yogurt or yogurt	175 mL
2 tbsp	grated orange zest	25 mL

1. In a medium bowl or plastic bag, combine sorghum flour, amaranth flour, brown rice flour, tapioca starch, sugar, xanthan gum, baking powder, baking soda, salt and nutmeg. Mix well and set aside.

2. In a large bowl, using an electric mixer, beat egg, egg white, pineapple, oil and vanilla until combined. Add yogurt and orange zest; mix just until combined. Add dry ingredients and mix just until combined.

3. Spoon batter evenly into each cup of prepared muffin tin. Let stand for 30 minutes. Meanwhile, preheat oven to 350°F (180°C).

4. Bake for 20 to 25 minutes, or until a tester comes out clean. Let cool in pan on a rack for 5 minutes.

> **To make this recipe egg-free**
> Omit egg and egg white from recipe. Add 1 tsp (5 mL) powdered egg replacer with the dry ingredients and add 2 tbsp (25 mL) water with the liquids.

**NUTRITIONAL VALUE
per serving**

Calories	161
Fat, total	6 g
Fat, saturated	1 g
Cholesterol	16 mg
Sodium	218 mg
Carbohydrate	24 g
Fiber	2 g
Protein	3 g
Calcium	53 mg
Iron	2 mg

Cookies, Squares and More

Oatmeal Raisin Cookies

Makes 54 cookies (1 per serving)

As with all true oatmeal raisin cookies, we find we have great difficulty sampling just one of these. The cover photo is enough to send us immediately to the kitchen to bake!

Tips

Underbake for a chewy cookie. Bake longer for a crisp one. Watch carefully, as cookies burn within an extra 1 to 2 minutes.

To make Oatmeal Raisin Bars, bake in a lightly greased 9-inch (2.5 L) baking pan for 25 minutes.

♦ *Preheat oven to 350°F (180°C)*
♦ *Baking sheets, lightly greased*

¾ cup	GF oat flour	175 mL
¼ cup	tapioca starch	50 mL
½ tsp	xanthan gum	2 mL
¾ tsp	baking soda	4 mL
¾ cup	lactose-free buttery spread or butter, softened	175 mL
½ cup	granulated sugar	125 mL
½ cup	packed brown sugar	125 mL
1	egg	1
2 tsp	vanilla	10 mL
2½ cups	GF oats	625 mL
1½ cups	raisins	375 mL

1. In a small bowl or plastic bag, combine oat flour, tapioca starch, xanthan gum and baking soda. Mix well and set aside.

2. In a large bowl, using an electric mixer, beat buttery spread, sugar, brown sugar, egg and vanilla until light and fluffy. Slowly beat in dry ingredients until combined. Stir in oats and raisins.

3. Drop dough by rounded spoonfuls 2 inches (5 cm) apart on prepared baking sheets.

4. Bake in preheated oven for 10 to 13 minutes, or until lightly browned and just set. Let cool on baking sheets on a rack for 2 to 3 minutes. Carefully transfer to a cooling rack and let cool completely. Store in an airtight container at room temperature for up to 5 days or freeze for up to 2 months.

> **To make this recipe egg-free**
> Omit egg from recipe. Combine 2 tbsp (25 mL) flax flour or ground flaxseed with ¼ cup (50 mL) warm water. Let stand for 5 minutes. Add with vanilla.

NUTRITIONAL VALUE
per serving

Calories	70
Fat, total	2 g
Fat, saturated	1 g
Cholesterol	4 mg
Sodium	34 mg
Carbohydrate	12 g
Fiber	1 g
Protein	1 g
Calcium	8 mg
Iron	1 mg

Peanut Butter Cookies

Makes 42 cookies (1 per serving)

Here's a much-requested recipe for those who can't have soy. These crunchy cookies are a delicious, nutritious addition to any lunch or snack.

Tips

If the dough sticks to the fork while flattening, dip fork into sweet rice flour.

For a crunchier cookie, substitute buttery spread or soft butter for the shortening.

Select a shortening that is low in trans fats, if available in your area. It will not affect measuring, taste or performance.

- ♦ *Preheat oven to 350°F (180°C)*
- ♦ *Baking sheets, lightly greased*

1 ¼ cups	amaranth flour	300 mL
¼ cup	cornstarch	50 mL
½ tsp	xanthan gum	2 mL
½ tsp	baking soda	2 mL
¼ tsp	salt	1 mL
¼ cup	shortening	50 mL
½ cup	smooth peanut butter	125 mL
1 cup	packed brown sugar	250 mL
½ tsp	vanilla	2 mL
1	egg	1

1. In a small bowl or plastic bag, combine amaranth flour, cornstarch, xanthan gum, baking soda and salt. Mix well and set aside.

2. In a large bowl, using an electric mixer, cream shortening, peanut butter and brown sugar. Add vanilla and egg; beat until well blended. Slowly beat in dry ingredients until just combined.

3. Roll into 1-inch (2.5 cm) balls. Place 2 inches (5 cm) apart on prepared baking sheet. Flatten slightly with a fork.

4. Bake in preheated oven for 10 to 12 minutes, or until set. Let cool on pan on a rack for 2 minutes. Transfer to a cooling rack and let cool completely. Store in an airtight container at room temperature for up to 5 days or freeze for up to 2 months.

To make this recipe egg-free

Omit egg from recipe. Combine 2 tbsp (25 mL) flax flour or ground flaxseed with ¼ cup (50 mL) warm water. Let stand for 5 minutes. Add with vanilla.

Variation

For a crisper cookie, bake the egg-free version.

NUTRITIONAL VALUE
per serving

Calories	67
Fat, total	3 g
Fat, saturated	1 g
Cholesterol	4 mg
Sodium	47 mg
Carbohydrate	9 g
Fiber	0 g
Protein	1 g
Calcium	11 mg
Iron	1 mg

Pumpkin Chocolate Chip Cookies

Makes 48 cookies (1 per serving)

Imagine a hermit cookie — soft, cake-like texture and pumpkin color with dots of chocolate.

Tips

Select good-quality chocolate chips. Read the label: chocolate liquor and cocoa butter should come before sugar in the list of ingredients.

For a crunchier cookie, substitute buttery spread or soft butter for the shortening.

Select a shortening that is low in trans fats, if available in your area. It will not affect measuring, taste or performance.

NUTRITIONAL VALUE per serving

Calories	80
Fat, total	4 g
Fat, saturated	1 g
Cholesterol	0 mg
Sodium	4 mg
Carbohydrate	11 g
Fiber	1 g
Protein	1 g
Calcium	19 mg
Iron	1 mg

♦ Baking sheets, lightly greased

1 cup	sorghum flour	250 mL
⅔ cup	whole bean flour	150 mL
½ cup	tapioca starch	125 mL
1 tsp	xanthan gum	5 mL
2 tsp	GF baking powder	10 mL
1 tsp	baking soda	5 mL
¼ tsp	salt	1 mL
2 tsp	ground cinnamon	10 mL
½ tsp	ground ginger	2 mL
1 cup	canned pumpkin purée (not pie filling)	250 mL
¾ cup	packed brown sugar	175 mL
½ cup	shortening	125 mL
2 tbsp	grated orange zest	25 mL
1½ cups	lactose-free chocolate chips or chocolate chips (see tip, at left)	375 mL

1. In a medium bowl or plastic bag, combine sorghum flour, whole bean flour, tapioca starch, xanthan gum, baking powder, baking soda, salt, cinnamon and ginger. Mix well and set aside.

2. In a large bowl, using an electric mixer, beat pumpkin purée, brown sugar and shortening for 3 minutes, until smooth. Slowly beat in dry ingredients until combined. Stir in orange zest and chocolate chips.

3. Drop dough by rounded spoonfuls 2 inches (5 cm) apart on prepared baking sheets. Flatten slightly with a fork. Let stand for 30 minutes. Meanwhile, preheat oven to 350°F (180°C).

4. Bake in preheated oven for 10 to 14 minutes, or until set. Transfer to a cooling rack and let cool completely. Store in an airtight container at room temperature for up to 5 days or freeze for up to 2 months.

Lacy Tuiles

Makes 8 cookies (1 per serving)

Tuile (pronounced *twee*) is the French word for "tile" and describes a thin, crisp wafer cookie traditionally shaped while still hot around a curved object such as a rolling pin.

Tips

Don't worry if wafers spread together during baking — just wait until they're cool and break apart.

The days we make Lime Sorbet (page 287), we freeze 2 tbsp (25 mL) of the extra coconut milk from the can for this recipe.

- ♦ *Preheat oven to 375°F (190°C)*
- ♦ *Large rimless baking sheets, lined with parchment paper*

2 tbsp	coconut milk	25 mL
¼ cup	granulated sugar	50 mL
1 tbsp	lactose-free margarine or margarine	15 mL
⅓ cup	unsweetened shredded coconut	75 mL
2 tbsp	tapioca starch	25 mL

1. In a microwave-safe bowl, combine coconut milk, sugar and margarine. Microwave on High for 30 to 60 seconds, or until sugar dissolves. Stir in coconut and tapioca starch.

2. Drop by tablespoonfuls (15 mL) at least 5 inches (12.5 cm) apart onto prepared baking sheets. Make only 4 at a time. Spread with the back of a spoon to a 3-inch (7.5 cm) circle to distribute coconut evenly.

3. Bake in center of preheated oven for 7 to 9 minutes, or until a dark caramel color, bubbly and lacy. (Watch carefully, as they brown quickly.) Let cool on pan on a rack for 2 minutes. Using a metal spatula or lifter, remove from baking sheets and place on paper towels. Cover with additional paper towels. Gently pat. Let cool completely between paper towels. Store between layers of waxed paper in an airtight container at room temperature for up to 3 days.

Variations

Let baked tuiles cool for 30 seconds. Then, while they're still warm and pliable, loosely roll wafer around the handle of a wooden spoon or rolling pin. Slip off and place on paper towels until completely cooled. If cookies become too crisp before all are rolled, place back in warm, but turned-off oven just until soft and pliable.

Drop batter by teaspoonfuls (5 mL) and spread to make 2 dozen mini Lacy Tuiles. Reduce baking time to 5 to 7 minutes, and watch carefully.

NUTRITIONAL VALUE per serving	
Calories	66
Fat, total	4 g
Fat, saturated	2 g
Cholesterol	0 mg
Sodium	16 mg
Carbohydrate	9 g
Fiber	1 g
Protein	0 g
Calcium	2 mg
Iron	0 mg

Orange Almond Strips

Makes 64 cookies (1 per serving)

A chewy cookie with a crunchy almond topping — we dare you to eat just one!

Tips

We used a 100% vegan, non-dairy buttery spread.

When using 2 jelly-roll pans, place them in the upper and lower thirds of the oven. Switch their positions and rotate back to front halfway through the baking time for even baking.

♦ *Preheat oven to 325°F (160°C)*
♦ *Two 15- by 10-inch (40 by 25 cm) jelly-roll pans, ungreased*

¾ cup	rice flour	175 mL
½ cup	almond flour	125 mL
¼ cup	soy flour	50 mL
¼ cup	cornstarch	50 mL
1 tsp	xanthan gum	5 mL
2 tsp	GF baking powder	10 mL
1 tbsp	grated orange zest	15 mL
½ cup	lactose-free buttery spread or butter, softened	125 mL
1 cup	granulated sugar	250 mL
1 tsp	almond extract	5 mL
1	egg	1
2 tbsp	fortified soy beverage, lactose-free milk or milk	25 mL
½ cup	sliced or chopped almonds	125 mL

1. In a medium bowl or plastic bag, combine rice flour, almond flour, soy flour, cornstarch, xanthan gum, baking powder and orange zest. Mix well and set aside.

2. In a large bowl, using an electric mixer, cream buttery spread, sugar, almond extract and egg until blended. (Mixture may appear curdled.) Slowly beat in dry ingredients until just combined.

3. Divide dough into 4 equal portions. Place 2 portions crosswise in each jelly-roll pan, leaving lots of room between them to allow for spreading. Using your hands, flatten each portion into an 8- by 2-inch (20 cm by 5 cm) rectangle. Brush each with soy beverage. Sprinkle each with one-quarter of the almonds, pressing in lightly.

NUTRITIONAL VALUE
per serving

Calories	40
Fat, total	2 g
Fat, saturated	0 g
Cholesterol	3 mg
Sodium	10 mg
Carbohydrate	6 g
Fiber	0 g
Protein	1 g
Calcium	13 mg
Iron	0 mg

Use a pizza wheel to make cutting the strips quick and easy.

4. Bake in preheated oven for 15 to 20 minutes, or until edges are light brown, rotating pans halfway through (see tip, page 272). Let cool slightly. Transfer to a cutting board. While still warm, cut each in half lengthwise, then crosswise into 2-inch (5 cm) wide strips. Transfer to a cooling rack and let cool completely. Store in an airtight container at room temperature for up to 5 days or freeze for up to 2 months.

To make this recipe egg-free
Omit egg from recipe. Add 1 tsp (5 mL) powdered egg replacer with the dry ingredients and add 2 tbsp (25 mL) water with the buttery spread.

Variation
If you like an iced cookie, in a small bowl, sift 1 cup (250 mL) GF confectioner's (icing) sugar. Stir in $\frac{1}{4}$ tsp (1 mL) almond extract and 1 to 2 tbsp (15 to 25 mL) freshly squeezed orange juice, adding just enough to thin icing to a drizzling consistency. Drizzle icing over cooled cookies.

Cherry Almond Biscotti

Makes 24 cookies (1 per serving)

Biscotti, a traditional Italian cookie, has become part of our Canadian cuisine. In this version, the tantalizing taste of sour cherries contrasts with the sweetness of almond. The picture of this cookie on the cover will whet your appetite!

Tips

For information on toasting nuts, see the Technique Glossary, page 301.

Biscotti will be medium-firm and crunchy. For softer, chewier biscotti, bake for only 10 minutes in Step 5; for very firm biscotti, bake for 20 minutes.

UTRITIONAL VALUE per serving	
Calories	76
Fat, total	3 g
Fat, saturated	0 g
Cholesterol	16 mg
Sodium	6 mg
Carbohydrate	11 g
Fiber	0 g
Protein	2 g
Calcium	25 mg
Iron	1 mg

+ *Preheat oven to 325°F (160°C)*
+ *8-inch (2 L) square baking pan, lightly greased*
+ *Baking sheets, ungreased*

¾ cup	amaranth flour	175 mL
¼ cup	almond flour	50 mL
3 tbsp	tapioca starch	45 mL
2 tbsp	cornstarch	25 mL
¾ tsp	xanthan gum	4 mL
½ tsp	GF baking powder	2 mL
Pinch	salt	Pinch
2	eggs	2
½ cup	granulated sugar	125 mL
½ tsp	almond extract	2 mL
¾ cup	sliced almonds, toasted	175 mL
½ cup	dried sour cherries	125 mL

1. In a small bowl or plastic bag, combine amaranth flour, almond flour, tapioca starch, cornstarch, xanthan gum, baking powder and salt. Mix well and set aside.

2. In a large bowl, using an electric mixer, beat eggs, sugar and almond extract until combined. Slowly beat in dry ingredients until just combined. Stir in almonds and cherries.

3. Spoon into prepared pan. Using a moistened rubber spatula, spread batter to edges and smooth top.

4. Bake in preheated oven for 30 to 35 minutes, or until firm and top is just turning golden. Let cool in pan for 5 minutes. Remove from pan and let cool on a cutting board for 5 minutes. Cut into quarters, then cut each quarter into 6 slices.

5. Arrange slices upright (both cut sides exposed) at least ½ inch (1 cm) apart on baking sheets. Bake for 15 minutes, until dry and crisp. Transfer to a cooling rack and let cool completely. Store in an airtight container at room temperature for up to 6 weeks or freeze for up to 6 months.

Tip

Recipe can be doubled. Use a 13- by 9-inch (3 L) baking pan and increase baking time in Step 4 by about 5 minutes, or use two 8-inch (2 L) pans.

To make this recipe egg-free

Omit eggs from recipe. Combine $\frac{1}{4}$ cup (50 mL) flax flour or ground flaxseed with $\frac{1}{2}$ cup (125 mL) warm water. Let stand 5 minutes. Add with the almond extract.

Variations

Substitute 1 tbsp (15 mL) grated lemon zest for the almond extract.

Substitute hazelnuts and hazelnut flour for the almonds and almond flour.

Carol's Brownies

Makes 18 large brownies (1 per serving)

Tips

The brownies look rather wet when baked, but don't increase the baking time.

Do not substitute high-fat soy flour or brownies won't bake as well.

Carol liked to use safflower oil as her vegetable oil.

♦ *Preheat oven to 350°F (180°C)*
♦ *13- by 9-inch (3 L) baking pan, lightly greased*

¾ cup	low-fat or defatted soy flour	175 mL
¾ cup	tapioca starch	175 mL
2 cups	granulated sugar	500 mL
½ cup	unsweetened cocoa powder, sifted	125 mL
½ tsp	GF baking powder	2 mL
¼ tsp	salt	1 mL
4	eggs	4
1 cup	vegetable oil	250 mL
¼ cup	water	50 mL
4 tsp	vanilla	20 mL

1. In a large bowl or plastic bag, combine soy flour, tapioca starch, sugar, cocoa, baking powder and salt. Mix well and set aside.

2. In a separate bowl, combine eggs, oil, water and vanilla until blended. Stir in dry ingredients until just combined.

3. Pour into prepared pan. Using a rubber spatula, spread to edges and smooth top.

4. Bake in preheated oven for 30 to 35 minutes, or until moist crumbs cling to a tester inserted in the center. Let cool completely in pan on a rack. Cut into bars. Store in an airtight container at room temperature for up to 5 days or freeze for up to 2 months.

Variations

Use your favourite chocolate frosting recipe to add extra pizzazz to these brownies. Be sure to use GF confectioner's (icing) sugar.

UTRITIONAL VALUE per serving	
Calories	248
Fat, total	14 g
Fat, saturated	1 g
Cholesterol	42 mg
Sodium	47 mg
Carbohydrate	30 g
Fiber	1 g
Protein	4 g
Calcium	25 mg
Iron	1 mg

A Family Favorite

We asked Gary, our dear friend Carol Coulter's non-celiac husband, for one of her favorite recipes to include in this book. He said, "We didn't have any trouble picking the brownie recipe because she would whip it up whenever family or friends were coming. I don't ever remember eating them frosted, as they didn't ever last that long. I think she did frost them if she took them 'out,' but here at home they were always eaten plain or with ice cream for dessert." Carol Coulter's daughter Pam says, "Mom's 'pressure-treated' brownies are better than any wheat flour brownie ever made!"

To learn more about our friend Carol, see page 12. This book is dedicated to her.

Carrot Pecan Hermit Bars

Makes 16 bars (1 per serving)

Hermit cookies have been around since the late 1800s. Here, we've adapted the traditional recipe into a soft, spicy, chewy bar. The ragged and speckled appearance reminds us of a hermit's robe.

Tip

The batter is very thick, so the moistened spatula is necessary to spread it evenly.

♦ 9-inch (2.5 L) square baking pan, lightly greased

⅔ cup	low-fat or defatted soy flour	150 mL
⅓ cup	quinoa flour	75 mL
2 tbsp	arrowroot starch	25 mL
½ cup	packed brown sugar	125 mL
1 tsp	xanthan gum	5 mL
1 tsp	GF baking powder	5 mL
½ tsp	salt	2 mL
½ tsp	ground cinnamon	2 mL
½ tsp	ground nutmeg	2 mL
¼ tsp	ground allspice	1 mL
¼ tsp	ground cloves	1 mL
1 tbsp	grated orange zest	15 mL
2	eggs	2
⅓ cup	vegetable oil	75 mL
1 tsp	vanilla	10 mL
1½ cups	shredded carrots	375 mL
¾ cup	dried cranberries	175 mL
¾ cup	chopped pecans	175 mL

1. In a medium bowl or plastic bag, combine soy flour, quinoa flour, arrowroot starch, brown sugar, xanthan gum, baking powder, salt, cinnamon, nutmeg, allspice, cloves and orange zest. Mix well and set aside.

2. In a large bowl, using a heavy-duty electric mixer with paddle attachment, beat eggs, oil and vanilla until blended. Slowly beat in dry ingredients until just combined. Stir in carrots, cranberries and pecans.

3. Spoon into prepared pan. Using a moistened rubber spatula, spread to edges and smooth top. Let stand for 30 minutes. Meanwhile preheat oven to 350°F (180°C).

4. Bake in preheated oven for 30 to 35 minutes, or until a cake tester inserted in the center comes out clean. Let cool completely in pan on a rack. Cut into bars. Layer bars between sheets of parchment or waxed paper in an airtight container and store at room temperature for up to 5 days or freeze for up to 2 months.

NUTRITIONAL VALUE per serving	
Calories	163
Fat, total	9 g
Fat, saturated	1 g
Cholesterol	23 mg
Sodium	88 mg
Carbohydrate	17 g
Fiber	2 g
Protein	4 g
Calcium	43 mg
Iron	1 mg

Tip

Grate carrots using the large holes of a box grater or the shredding blade of a food processor. Any extra grated carrot can be added to a salad. One large carrot yields about 1 cup (250 mL) grated.

To make this recipe egg-free
Omit eggs from recipe. Combine ¼ cup (50 mL) flax flour or ground flaxseed with ½ cup (125 mL) warm water. Let stand for 5 minutes. Add with vanilla.

Variations

Substitute raisins for the cranberries and/or walnuts for the pecans

Substitute dates, apricots or unsweetened shredded coconut for either the cranberries or the pecans.

Purchasing Pecans

A fresh crop of pecans arrives in the stores in November each year. Shells should crack easily and release most of the kernel (nut meat) in one or more large pieces. The kernel should be a very light color, without stains or dark spots, and the texture should be crisp, not soft (green) or brittle (old). There should be no hint of bitterness in the flavor. Pecans can be purchased in the shell or shelled. Shelled nuts are sold in perfect halves or in pieces, granules or meal. Purchase plump nuts that are uniform in color and size. Pieces are usually less expensive.

- 1 lb (450 g) in-shell pecans yields 8 to 9 oz (240 to 270 g) pecan halves.
- 1 cup (250 mL) chopped pecans weighs 5 oz (150 g).

Oatmeal Mincemeat Squares

Makes 16 squares (1 per serving)

A quick and easy snacking bar — just use the same mixture for the crust and topping and a store-bought mincemeat for the filling.

Tips

For information about GF oat flakes and GF oat flour, see pages 37–39.

Recipe can easily be doubled and baked in a 13- by 9-inch (3 L) baking pan for 40 to 45 minutes.

Squares are delicious served warm for dessert. If serving as a dessert, cut into 9 larger squares.

♦ *Preheat oven to 350°F (180°C)*
♦ *8-inch (2 L) square baking pan, lightly greased*

1⅓ cups	GF oat flakes	325 mL
⅔ cup	amaranth flour	150 mL
⅔ cup	GF oat flour	150 mL
⅔ cup	granulated sugar	150 mL
¼ tsp	baking soda	1 mL
¼ tsp	salt	1 mL
½ cup	lactose-free buttery spread or butter, melted	125 mL
1 cup	GF mincemeat	250 mL

1. In a large bowl, combine oats, amaranth flour, oat flour, sugar, baking soda and salt. Mix well. Stir in melted buttery spread until mixture is soft and crumbly.

2. Reserve 1 cup (250 mL) of crumb mixture for topping. Firmly pat the remaining mixture into prepared pan. Spread mincemeat evenly over base and sprinkle with reserved crumb mixture. Do not press mixture down; it should be crumbly on top.

3. Bake in preheated oven for 30 to 35 minutes, or until light golden brown. Let cool completely in pan on a rack. Cut into squares. Store in an airtight container in the refrigerator for up to 5 days or freeze for up to 2 months.

NUTRITIONAL VALUE per serving	
Calories	174
Fat, total	4 g
Fat, saturated	1 g
Cholesterol	0 mg
Sodium	116 mg
Carbohydrate	31 g
Fiber	2 g
Protein	3 g
Calcium	15 mg
Iron	3 mg

Variations

If you are unable to tolerate oats, substitute buckwheat, quinoa or amaranth flakes for the GF oat flakes and sorghum flour for the oat flour.

Oatmeal Berry Squares: Substitute berry jam for the GF mincemeat. We used a sugar-reduced mixed berry jam. If you use a full-sugar jam, reduce the sugar in the recipe to ½ cup (125 mL).

Halvah

Makes 18 bars (1 per serving)

Halvah (or halva) is a Middle Eastern confection made from ground sesame seeds and honey. Ours is spiced, but it is sometimes flavored with nuts, dried fruit and chocolate. Enjoy as a snack.

Tips

For fast, easy cutting, use a pizza wheel.

Pulsing half the sesame seeds first gives a crunchier halvah.

- Preheat oven to 350°F (180°C)
- 9-inch (2.5 L) square baking pan, lightly greased and lined with parchment paper

2 cups	sesame seeds, divided	500 mL
¼ cup	liquid honey	50 mL
½ tsp	ground allspice	2 mL
½ tsp	ground cinnamon	2 mL
½ tsp	ground ginger	2 mL

1. In a food processor fitted with a metal blade, process 1 cup (250 mL) of the sesame seeds, scraping down sides with a rubber spatula once or twice, for 2 to 3 minutes, or until seeds form a coarse paste. Add the remaining sesame seeds, honey, allspice, cinnamon and ginger; pulse until just blended (do not over-process).

2. Pat into prepared pan and bake in preheated oven for 11 to 13 minutes, or until lightly browned. Let cool in pan on a rack for 5 minutes. Remove from pan and cut into bars while still warm. Let cool completely on rack. Store in an airtight container at room temperature for up to 5 days or freeze for up to 2 months.

Variation

Omit allspice, cinnamon and ginger and add 1 cup (250 mL) of a combination of chopped dried fruit, nuts and lactose-free chocolate chips or chocolate chips.

NUTRITIONAL VALUE per serving

Calories	107
Fat, total	8 g
Fat, saturated	1 g
Cholesterol	0 mg
Sodium	2 mg
Carbohydrate	8 g
Fiber	2 g
Protein	3 g
Calcium	158 mg
Iron	2 mg

Shirley's Old-Fashioned Donuts

Makes 20 donuts (1 per serving)

We've had many requests for donut recipes, so when our celiac friend Shirley offered us hers, we jumped at it. These old-fashioned cake donuts have just the right hint of cinnamon and nutmeg. Enjoy them warm.

Tips

See the Equipment Glossary, pages 291–292, for information on donut cutters and thermometers.

For information on potato flour, see pages 55 and 56.

Recipe can be doubled.

- Deep fryer or deep saucepan
- Candy/fat thermometer
- 2¼-inch (6 cm) donut cutter

½ cup	fortified soy beverage, lactose-free milk or milk	125 mL
1 tsp	freshly squeezed lemon juice	5 mL
½ cup	whole bean flour	125 mL
¼ cup	sorghum flour	50 mL
⅔ cup	tapioca starch	150 mL
½ cup	cornstarch	125 mL
1 tbsp	potato flour (*not* potato starch)	15 mL
2 tsp	xanthan gum	10 mL
1¼ tsp	baking soda	6 mL
1¼ tsp	cream of tartar	6 mL
Pinch	salt	Pinch
¼ tsp	ground cinnamon	1 mL
¼ tsp	ground nutmeg	1 mL
1	egg	1
½ cup	granulated sugar	125 mL
2 tbsp	vegetable oil	25 mL
¼ tsp	vanilla	1 mL
	Vegetable oil for frying	
	Sweet rice flour	

1. In a liquid measuring cup or bowl, combine soy beverage and lemon juice; set aside for 5 minutes.
2. Meanwhile, in a medium bowl or plastic bag, combine whole bean flour, sorghum flour, tapioca starch, cornstarch, potato flour, xanthan gum, baking soda, cream of tartar, salt, cinnamon and nutmeg. Mix well and set aside.
3. In a large bowl, using an electric mixer, beat egg, sugar, oil, vanilla and soy beverage mixture until blended. Add dry ingredients and mix until combined.

NUTRITIONAL VALUE per serving	
Calories	81
Fat, total	2 g
Fat, saturated	0 g
Cholesterol	10 mg
Sodium	101 mg
Carbohydrate	16 g
Fiber	1 g
Protein	1 g
Calcium	18 mg
Iron	0 mg

Tips

Cut as many donuts as possible the first time you roll out the dough. Scraps require chilling before they can be rerolled.

As these donuts brown quickly, we always measure the thickness of the rolled-out dough with a ruler. If donuts are too thick, they get brown before the center cooks.

If dough becomes sticky when rolling and cutting, return to the refrigerator for a few minutes.

While still warm, dust donuts with sifted GF confectioner's (icing) sugar or cinnamon-sugar.

4. Divide dough in half. Place each half between two sheets of plastic wrap and pat out to a disk about $\frac{1}{2}$ inch (1 cm) thick. Wrap airtight and refrigerate overnight.

5. Preheat $1\frac{1}{2}$ to 2 inches (3 to 5 cm) of oil in a deep fryer or a deep saucepan to 350°F (180°C), keeping a close eye on the temperature. Meanwhile, remove one disk of dough from the refrigerator. Place between 2 clean sheets of plastic wrap and roll out to $\frac{1}{4}$-inch (0.5 cm) thickness. Cut with donut cutter, chilling and rerolling scraps. (If dough sticks to cutter, dip cutter into sweet rice flour.)

6. Deep-fry donuts, a few at a time, for 15 to 20 seconds on each side, or until golden brown. Drain on paper towels. Repeat with remaining dough. Store in an airtight container at room temperature for up to 2 days or freeze for up to 2 months.

> **To make this recipe egg-free**
> Omit egg from recipe. Combine 2 tbsp (25 mL) flax flour or ground flaxseed with $\frac{1}{4}$ cup (50 mL) warm water. Let stand for 5 minutes. Add with vanilla.

> When Shirley Stewart adapted this recipe to gluten-free, she researched its origin. The original wheat flour version, which her mother-in-law and sister-in-law have used for years, came from an early 1900s cookbook compiled by the Upper Musquodoboit Women's Institute in Nova Scotia. The recipe was submitted by Mrs. A.D. Burris, a distant relative of Shirley's. The original recipe used 4 cups (1 L) of all-purpose flour, and used lard to fry the donuts. We've adapted it for you!

Apricot Pear Pudding

Makes 4 servings

Enjoy this versatile dessert when you come home from walking the dog on a cold winter night.

Tips

Pears ripen from the inside out and can spoil very quickly, especially if left at room temperature too long. To check for ripeness, gently press the stem end; it will yield slightly when ripe. Pears are very high in fiber, so enjoy them often.

♦

To turn this pudding into a sauce, decrease the cornstarch to 2 tsp (10 mL). Omit the crust and serve warm over a white or gingerbread cake.

♦ Four ¾-cup (175 mL) ramekins or soufflé dishes

Crust

¾ cup	Gingerbread Crumbs (see recipe, page 238)	175 mL
1 tbsp	lactose-free buttery spread or butter, melted	15 mL

Pudding

1½ cups	pear juice	375 mL
½ cup	dried apricots, quartered	125 mL
2	pears	2
¼ cup	granulated sugar	50 mL
2 tbsp	cornstarch	25 mL
2 tbsp	freshly squeezed lemon juice	25 mL

1. *Prepare the crust:* In a small bowl, combine Gingerbread Crumbs and buttery spread. Press 2 tbsp (25 mL) into the bottom of each ramekin. Reserve the remaining crumbs for topping. Set dishes aside.

2. *Prepare the pudding:* In a medium saucepan, over medium-high heat, bring pear juice and apricots to a boil. Reduce heat to low and simmer gently for 10 minutes, or until apricots are tender.

3. Meanwhile, peel pears and cut in half lengthwise. Remove stems and cores and cut each half into eighths. Set aside.

4. In a small bowl, combine sugar and cornstarch; stir in lemon juice until blended. Stir into apricot mixture, then stir in pears. Cook over medium-high heat, stirring constantly, until mixture comes to a boil. Reduce heat to low and simmer gently, stirring constantly, for 2 to 3 minutes, or until pudding becomes thick and shiny.

5. Spoon pudding over crust in ramekins. Sprinkle with remaining crumbs. Refrigerate for at least 1 hour.

NUTRITIONAL VALUE per serving

Calories	322
Fat, total	8 g
Fat, saturated	2 g
Cholesterol	0 mg
Sodium	101 mg
Carbohydrate	62 g
Fiber	3 g
Protein	2 g
Calcium	52 mg
Iron	2 mg

Variation

Add ¼ cup (50 mL) dried cranberries with the pears.

Baked Apples

Makes 6 servings

Here's a modern twist on an old favorite — still warming and welcoming on a cold winter's night.

Tips

Use either an apple corer or a melon baller to scoop out the core from the apple.

If your baking dish doesn't have a lid, cover it with aluminum foil.

Use your favorite baking apple variety. We like Spartan, Cortland, Crispin (Mutsu), Golden Delicious, Granny Smith, Ida Red, Jonagold, Northern Spy or Braeburn.

For information on toasting nuts, see the Technique Glossary, page 301.

NUTRITIONAL VALUE per serving	
Calories	475
Fat, total	16 g
Fat, saturated	3 g
Cholesterol	0 mg
Sodium	63 mg
Carbohydrate	85 g
Fiber	9 g
Protein	4 g
Calcium	74 mg
Iron	3 mg

◆ *Preheat oven to 375°F (190°C)*
◆ *11- by 8½-inch (2.5 L) oval glass baking dish with lid*

Syrup

1 cup	apple cider	250 mL
⅔ cup	pure maple syrup or maple-flavored syrup	150 mL
1 tbsp	lactose-free buttery spread or butter	15 mL
1 cup	Streusel Topping (see recipe, page 290)	250 mL
½ cup	dried cranberries	125 mL
½ cup	snipped dried apricots	125 mL
½ cup	chopped toasted pecans	125 mL
½ tsp	ground cinnamon	2 mL
½ tsp	ground nutmeg	2 mL
6	large baking apples	6
2 tbsp	brandy (optional)	25 mL

1. *Prepare the syrup:* In a medium saucepan, combine cider, maple syrup and buttery spread. Bring to a boil, stirring frequently. Reduce heat to medium-low and simmer for 10 minutes. Set aside.

2. In a medium bowl, combine streusel topping, cranberries, apricots, pecans, cinnamon and nutmeg. Set aside.

3. Core each apple, making at least a 1-inch (2.5 cm) diameter cavity in the center and leaving the bottom intact. Halfway down from the top of each apple, using a paring knife or vegetable peeler, remove a 1-inch (2.5 cm) wide strip of peel. Place apples upright in baking dish.

4. Pack streusel mixture into apple cavities, mounding excess on top and around sides. Pour syrup over apples and cover dish.

5. Bake in preheated oven for 20 minutes. Uncover, baste with syrup and drizzle with brandy, if using. Bake, uncovered, for 20 minutes, or until filling is crisp on top and apples are tender. Serve warm.

Caramelized Pears

Makes 4 servings

When the whole basket of pears finally ripens all at once, prepare this quick, easy, tasty dessert.

Tips

Place pears in a paper bag and keep at room temperature until ripe.

To test pears for ripeness, press lightly at the stem end; it should give slightly.

Choose firm pears that hold up well in cooking, such as Bartlett or Bosc.

♦ *Preheat oven to 400°F (200°C)*

♦ *9-inch (2.5 L) square or round glass, silicone or stoneware baking dish*

¼ cup	granulated sugar	50 mL
4	pears	4
1⅓ cups	pear juice	325 mL
1 tbsp	grated lemon zest	15 mL
¼ cup	freshly squeezed lemon juice	50 mL
½ cup	Streusel Topping (see recipe, page 290)	125 mL

1. Sprinkle sugar over bottom of baking dish.

2. Peel pears and cut in half lengthwise. Remove stems and cores. Trim a thin slice from the rounded side of each pear half to allow it to lie flat (when turning partway through baking). Place pears, rounded side up, on top of sugar.

3. In a small bowl, combine pear juice, lemon zest and lemon juice. Pour over pears.

4. Bake in preheated oven for 30 minutes, basting every 10 minutes. Turn pears over. Bake for 5 to 10 minutes, or until pears are fork-tender. Let cool in liquid. Meanwhile, preheat broiler.

5. Sprinkle streusel topping into the cavity of each pear half. Broil until pears are golden-brown. Place two pear halves on each of four dessert plates. Spoon remaining juice over pears.

Variations

Use fresh peaches instead of pears and reduce baking time by 5 to 10 minutes.

Substitute cranberry or pineapple juice for the pear juice.

Substitute Gingerbread Crumbs (page 238) for the Streusel Topping.

NUTRITIONAL VALUE per serving	
Calories	246
Fat, total	6 g
Fat, saturated	1 g
Cholesterol	0 mg
Sodium	36 mg
Carbohydrate	50 g
Fiber	4 g
Protein	2 g
Calcium	42 mg
Iron	2 mg

Lime Sorbet with Tropical Fruit and Lacy Tuiles

Makes 4 servings

This refreshing sorbet can be served on its own or combined with fruit and Lacy Tuiles (page 271) as a great make-ahead dessert for entertaining!

Tips

The sorbet recipe can be easily doubled; use a 9-inch (2.5 L) cake pan.

Sorbet will freeze more quickly in a metal pan than it will in a glass pan.

If sorbet is too firm to scoop, soften slightly in the refrigerator for up to 30 minutes.

Use an ice cream maker to freeze the sorbet. Follow the manufacturer's instructions.

NUTRITIONAL VALUE per serving

Calories	314
Fat, total	10 g
Fat, saturated	9 g
Cholesterol	0 mg
Sodium	30 mg
Carbohydrate	59 g
Fiber	5 g
Protein	3 g
Calcium	79 mg
Iron	3 mg

♦ 9- by 5-inch (2 L) loaf pan

Lime Sorbet

1	can (14 oz/400 mL) coconut milk	1
½ cup	granulated sugar	125 mL
2 tbsp	grated lime zest	25 mL
½ cup	freshly squeezed lime juice	125 mL
2 cups	pineapple spears	500 mL
3	kiwis, peeled and sliced	3
1	mango, peeled, pitted and sliced	1
	Lacy Tuiles (see recipe, page 271)	

1. Before opening can, shake coconut milk well to mix contents. Set aside 2 tbsp (25 mL) coconut milk to use in making Lacy Tuiles.
2. *Prepare the sorbet:* In a medium saucepan, over medium heat, heat coconut milk, sugar, lime zest and lime juice, stirring constantly, until sugar dissolves.
3. Pour into loaf pan and let cool completely. Freeze for 1½ to 2 hours, or until almost solid. Break up into chunks.
4. Transfer to a food processor and purée until smooth. Scrape into an airtight container and freeze for at least 4 hours, or until firm.
5. Arrange pineapple, kiwi and mango on chilled plates. Spoon sorbet beside fruit and garnish with Lacy Tuiles.

Variation

For a more decadent dessert, drizzle sorbet and fruit with Orange Sauce (page 263).

Mango Purée

2	very ripe large mangoes, peeled, pitted and cut into cubes	2
1 cup	water	250 mL
3 tbsp	granulated sugar	45 mL
2 tsp	freshly squeezed lime juice	10 mL

The rich flavor and color of mangoes takes a dessert from simple to exotic. Drizzle purée over lactose-free GF ice cream, Mango and Ginger Cream Tart (page 246), Date Orange Streusel Cake (page 264) or Lime Sorbet with Tropical Fruit and Lacy Tuiles (page 287). We also enjoy it with Chocolate Banana Snacking Cake (page 258) and Chocolate Ginger Cake (page 257).

Tip

For information on mangoes, see page 247.

1. In a large saucepan, combine mangoes, water, sugar and lime juice. Bring to a boil over medium-high heat, stirring frequently. Reduce heat to medium-low and simmer, stirring frequently, for 15 to 20 minutes, or until mangoes are soft.

2. Transfer to a blender or food processor and purée until smooth. Store in an airtight container in the refrigerator for up to 2 days.

Variations

Substitute fresh lemon juice for the lime and 4 large peaches for the mangoes.

Add 2 tbsp (25 mL) white rum to the purée just before serving.

NUTRITIONAL VALUE per serving

Calories	70
Fat, total	0 g
Fat, saturated	0 g
Cholesterol	0 mg
Sodium	3 mg
Carbohydrate	18 g
Fiber	1 g
Protein	0 g
Calcium	8 mg
Iron	0 mg

Harvest Compote

Makes 3 cups (750 mL) (½ cup/125 mL per serving)

1 cup	freshly squeezed orange juice	250 mL
¼ cup	granulated sugar	50 mL
1	cinnamon stick	1
3	apples (different varieties, see below), cored and coarsely chopped	3
½ cup	dried apricots, quartered	125 mL
½ cup	dried prunes, quartered	125 mL

Dried and fresh fruits cooked in an orange-flavored sugar syrup — what could be simpler? Serve this compote over GF Angel Food Cake (such as our version in *125 Best Gluten-Free Recipes*), lactose-free GF ice cream or lactose-free yogurt. You'll love the way the sweetness of the apples contrasts with the tanginess of the apricots and prunes.

1. In a large saucepan, combine orange juice, sugar and cinnamon stick. Heat over medium heat, stirring constantly, until sugar dissolves. Add apples, apricots and prunes; bring to a gentle boil. Reduce heat to low and simmer gently for 10 to 15 minutes, or until apples are fork-tender. Remove from heat and discard cinnamon stick. Transfer to a bowl, cover and refrigerate overnight.

Tips

There's no need to peel the apples.

Roll the orange, brought to room temperature, on the counter or between your hands for more juice.

Variation

For a stronger cinnamon flavor, leave the cinnamon stick in while the compote is chilling.

Using three kinds of apples gives the compote an interesting blend of flavors. Use your favorite baking apple varieties, but make sure to choose those that hold their shape. We like Spartan, Cortland, Crispin (Mutsu), Golden Delicious, Granny Smith, Ida Red, Jonagold, Northern Spy or Braeburn.

NUTRITIONAL VALUE per serving	
Calories	162
Fat, total	1 g
Fat, saturated	0 g
Cholesterol	0 mg
Sodium	2 mg
Carbohydrate	41 g
Fiber	3 g
Protein	1 g
Calcium	28 mg
Iron	1 mg

Streusel Topping

Makes 2½ cups (625 mL) (¼ cup/50 mL per serving)

This all-purpose topping can be used in a multitude of dishes. We've used it in Baked Apples (page 285) and Caramelized Pears (page 286). Try it sprinkled over lactose-free GF ice cream.

Tip

The mixture continues baking and browning when removed from the oven, so take it out before it gets dark.

♦ Preheat oven to 325°F (160°C)
♦ 15- by 10-inch (40 by 25 cm) jelly-roll pan

½ cup	almond flour	125 mL
½ cup	amaranth flour	125 mL
½ cup	cold lactose-free buttery spread or butter, cut into 1-inch (2.5 cm) cubes	125 mL
¼ cup	granulated sugar	50 mL
½ cup	slivered almonds, toasted	125 mL

1. In a food processor fitted with a metal blade, pulse almond flour, amaranth flour, buttery spread and sugar 5 to 7 times, or just until crumbly. Don't over-pulse. Add almonds and pulse just to mix. Transfer to jelly-roll pan, spreading out to a thin layer.

2. Bake in preheated oven for 10 minutes. Stir and bake for 5 minutes, or until a light golden brown. Let cool completely in pan on a rack. Store in an airtight container at room temperature for up to 1 month or freeze for up to 6 months.

Variation

Substitute coarsely chopped hazelnuts and hazelnut flour for the almonds and almond flour.

NUTRITIONAL VALUE
per serving

Calories	143
Fat, total	11 g
Fat, saturated	2 g
Cholesterol	0 mg
Sodium	52 mg
Carbohydrate	11 g
Fiber	2 g
Protein	3 g
Calcium	35 mg
Iron	2 mg

Equipment Glossary

Cake tester. A thin, long wooden or metal stick or wire attached to a handle, used for baked products to test for doneness.

Colander. A bowl-shaped utensil with many holes, used to drain liquids from solids.

Cooling rack. Parallel and perpendicular thin bars of metal at right angles, with feet attached, used to hold hot baking off the surface to allow cooling air to circulate.

Donut cutter. A utensil made of two 1-inch (2.5 cm) high rings, the smaller one centered inside the larger one. A U-shaped handle holds the rings together.

Grill. Heavy rack set over a heat source, used to cook food, usually on a propane, natural gas or charcoal barbecue.

Jelly-roll pan. A rectangular baking pan, 15 by 10 by 1 inch (40 by 25 by 2.5 cm), used for baking thin cakes.

Loaf pan. Container used for baking loaves. Common pan sizes are 9 by 5 inches (2 L) and 8 by 4 inches (1.5 L).

Mandolin(e). A manually operated slicer with adjustable blades. The food is held at a 45-degree angle and is passed and pressed against the blade to produce uniform pieces of different thickness, either straight-cut or rippled.

Mezzaluna. A two-handled knife with one or more thick, crescent-shaped blades (*mezzaluna* is Spanish for "half moon"). Used to chop or mince herbs and vegetables. Also known as a mincing knife.

OXO angled measuring cups. Made to give an accurate measure while set on the counter. There's no need to hold the measuring cup at eye level — you can look straight down as you fill it, and the angled insert lets you know when it is full enough. These cups are dishwasher-safe, but not microwaveable. Sizes available include $\frac{1}{4}$ cup (50 mL), 1 cup (250 mL), 2 cups (500 mL) and 4 cups (1 L). All sizes indicate metric and imperial amounts.

Paella pan. A wide shallow pan with gently sloping sides and two handles, often made of metal or earthenware.

Parchment paper. Heat-resistant paper similar to waxed paper, usually coated with silicon on one side; used with or as an alternative to other methods (such as applying vegetable oil or spray) to prevent baked goods from sticking to the baking pan. Sometimes labeled "baking paper."

Pastry blender. Used to cut solid fat into flour, it consists of five or six metal blades or wires held together by a handle.

Pastry brush. Small brush with nylon or natural bristles used to apply glazes or egg washes to dough. Wash thoroughly after each use. To store, lay flat or hang on a hook through the hole in the handle.

Pizza wheel. A sharp-edged wheel (without serrations) anchored to a handle.

Portion scoop. A utensil similar to an ice cream scoop, used to measure equal amounts of batter. Cookie scoops come in different sizes, for 2-inch (5 cm), $2\frac{1}{2}$-inch (6 cm) and $3\frac{1}{4}$-inch (8 cm) cookies. Muffin scoops have a $\frac{1}{4}$-cup (50 mL) capacity.

Ramekins. Usually sold as a set of small, deep, straight-sided ceramic soufflé dishes also known as mini bakers. Used to bake individual servings of a pudding, cobbler or custard. Capacity ranges from 4 oz, or $\frac{1}{2}$ cup (125 mL), to 8 oz, or 1 cup (250 mL).

Rolling pin. A smooth cylinder of wood, marble, plastic or metal; used to roll out dough.

Santoku knife. A knife with a flat edge that curves down near the point to a tip angle of around 60 degrees. It looks like a narrow-bladed cleaver and ranges from 5 to 8 inches (12.5 to 20 cm) in length. The blade has hollow recesses, called grantons, which create small air pockets between the blade and the food being sliced to keep it from sticking.

Sieve. A bowl-shaped utensil with many holes, used to drain liquids from solids.

Skewer. A long, thin stick (made of wood or metal) used in baking to test for doneness.

Spatula. A utensil with a handle and a blade that can be long or short, narrow or wide, flexible or inflexible. It is used to spread, lift, turn, mix or smooth foods. Spatulas are made of metal, rubber, plastic or silicone.

Springform pan. A circular baking pan, available in a range of sizes, with a separable bottom and side. The side is removed by releasing a clamp, making the contents easy to serve.

Thermometers.

- *Candy/fat thermometer.* Used to test the temperature of candy syrup or hot oil. Temperatures range from 75°F (25°C) to 400°F (200°C). A metal clip fastens to the side of the cooking pot, holding the tip of the thermometer off the bottom.

- *Instant-read thermometer.* Bakers use this metal-stemmed instrument to test the internal temperature of baked products such as cakes and breads. Stem must be inserted at least 2 inches (5 cm) into the food for an accurate reading. When yeast bread is baked, it should register 200°F (100°C).

- *Meat thermometer.* Used to read internal temperature of meat. Temperatures range from 120°F to 200°F (60°C to 100°C). Before placing meat in the oven, insert the thermometer into the thickest part, avoiding the bone and gristle. (If using an instant-read thermometer, remove meat from oven and test with thermometer. For more information, see Digital instant-read thermometer in the Technique Glossary, page 299.)

- *Oven thermometer.* Used to measure temperatures from 200°F to 500°F (100°C to 260°C). It either stands on or hangs from an oven rack.

Zester. A tool used to cut very thin strips of outer peel from citrus fruits. One type has a short, flat blade tipped with five small holes with sharp edges. Another style of zester that is popular is made of stainless steel and looks like a tool used for planing wood in a workshop.

Ingredient Glossary

Almonds. See "The Gluten-Free Pantry," page 34.

Almond flour (almond meal). See "The Gluten-Free Pantry," page 36.

Amaranth flour. See "The Gluten-Free Pantry," page 19.

Apricots. A small stone fruit with a thin, pale yellow to orange skin and meaty orange flesh. Dried unpeeled apricot halves are used in baking.

Arborio rice. See "The Gluten-Free Pantry," page 44.

Arrowroot. See "The Gluten-Free Pantry," page 54.

Baking chips. Similar in consistency to chocolate chips, but with different flavors such as butterscotch, peanut butter, cinnamon and lemon. Check to make sure they are gluten-free and lactose-free.

Baking powder. A chemical leavener, containing an alkali (baking soda) and an acid (cream of tartar), that gives off carbon dioxide gas under certain conditions. Select gluten-free baking powder.

Baking soda (sodium bicarbonate). A chemical leavener that gives off carbon dioxide gas in the presence of moisture — particularly acids such as lemon juice, buttermilk and sour cream. It is also one of the components of baking powder.

Balsamic vinegar. A dark Italian vinegar made from grape juice that has been cooked until the water content is reduced by half, then aged for several years in wooden barrels. It has a pungent sweetness and can be used to make salad dressings and marinades or drizzled over roasted or grilled vegetables.

Bean flours. See "The Gluten-Free Pantry," page 30.

Bell peppers. The sweet-flavored members of the capsicum family (which includes chilies and other hot peppers), these peppers have a hollow interior lined with white ribs and seeds attached at the stem end. They are most commonly green, red, orange or yellow, but can also be white or purple.

Blueberries. Wild low-bush berries are smaller than the cultivated variety and more time-consuming to pick, but their flavor makes every minute of picking time worthwhile. Readily available year-round in the frozen fruit section of most grocery stores.

Brown rice flour. See "The Gluten-Free Pantry," page 46.

Brown sugar. A refined sugar with a coating of molasses. It can be purchased coarse or fine and comes in three varieties: dark, golden and light.

Buckwheat. See "The Gluten-Free Pantry," page 21.

Butter. A spread produced from dairy fat and milk solids, butter is interchangeable with shortening, oil or margarine in most recipes. See also "Lactose Intolerance," page 62.

Buttery spread. See "Lactose Intolerance," page 64.

Capers. A pickled bud of the caper bush, grown in Mediterranean countries. Purchase in grocery stores in 2- to 3-oz (60 to 90 g) glass jars to use in sauces and salads and to enhance the flavor of smoked salmon.

Cardamom. This popular spice is a member of the ginger family. A long green or brown pod contains the strong, spicy, lemon-flavored seed. Although native to India, cardamom is used in Middle Eastern, Indian and Scandinavian cooking — in the latter case, particularly for seasonal baked goods.

Cassava. The plant from which tapioca comes.

Celery seeds. Small, light brown to khaki-colored seeds with an aroma similar to celery stalks. Their flavor is strong and bitter, and lingers on the palate.

Cheese, lactose-free. See "Lactose Intolerance," page 64.

Cilantro. See Coriander.

Coconut. The fruit of a tropical palm tree, with a hard woody shell that is lined with a hard white flesh. There are three dried forms available, which can be sweetened or not: flaked, shredded and the smallest, desiccated (thoroughly dried).

Coconut milk. A white liquid made by pouring boiling water over shredded coconut; the mixture is then cooled and strained.

Coriander. These tiny, yellow-ridged seeds taste of cardamom, cloves, white pepper and orange. Coriander leaves (also known as cilantro) have a flavor reminiscent of lemon, sage and caraway. To increase flavor in a recipe, substitute cilantro for parsley.

Corn flour. See "The Gluten-Free Pantry," page 24.

Cornmeal. See "The Gluten-Free Pantry," page 23.

Cornstarch. See "The Gluten-Free Pantry," page 55.

Corn syrup. A thick, sweet syrup made from cornstarch, sold in clear (light) or brown (dark or golden) varieties. The latter has caramel flavor and color added.

Cranberries. Grown in bogs on low vines, these sweet-tart berries are available fresh, frozen and dried. Fresh cranberries are available only in season — typically from mid-October until January, depending on your location — but can be frozen right in the bag. Substitute dried cranberries for sour cherries, raisins or currants.

Cream cheese, lactose-free. See "Lactose Intolerance," page 64.

Cream of tartar. Used to give volume and stability to beaten egg whites, cream of tartar is also an acidic component of baking powder. Tartaric acid is a fine white crystalline powder that forms naturally during the fermentation of grape juice on the inside of wine barrels.

Currants. Similar in appearance to small dark raisins, currants are made by drying a special seedless variety of grape. Not the same as a type of berry that goes by the same name.

Curry pastes. Mixtures of freshly ground whole dry spices with vegetable oil, garlic, and often other flavorings, such as lime peel, added. Pastes give a fuller, more aromatic flavor to a dish than most commercial curry powders do. In Thai cooking, there are many types of curry pastes, including orange and yellow, but red and green are the most common. Green pastes, made from fresh green chili peppers, are the hottest and are mainly used in poultry dishes. Red pastes, also searing hot, come from dried red chilies and are often used in beef curries or dishes that need a strong flavor. Check any curry paste to be sure it is gluten-free.

Dates. The fruit of the date palm tree, dates are long and oval in shape, with a paper-thin skin that turns from green to dark brown when ripe. Eaten fresh or dried, dates have a very sweet, light brown flesh around a long, narrow seed.

Egg replacer. See "Egg-Free Baking," page 66.

Eggs. Liquid egg products, such as Naturegg Simply Whites, Break-Free and Omega Pro liquid eggs and Just Whites, are available in the United States and Canada. Powdered egg whites such as Just Whites can be used by reconstituting with warm water or as a powder. A similar product is called meringue powder in Canada. Substitute 2 tbsp (25 mL) liquid egg product for each white of a large egg.

Fava bean flour. See "The Gluten-Free Pantry," page 30.

Fennel. A broad bulb with pale green celery-like stalks and bright green feathery leaves. The flavor is similar to anise, but sweeter and more delicate.

Feta cheese. A crumbly white Greek-style cheese with a salty, tangy flavor. Store in the refrigerator, in its brine, and drain well before using. Traditionally made with sheep's or goat's milk in Greece and usually with cow's milk in Canada and the U.S. A lactose-free flavored soy product is also available.

Fig. A pear-shaped fruit with a thick, soft skin, available in green and purple. Eaten fresh or dried, the tan-colored sweet flesh contains many tiny edible seeds.

Filberts. See Hazelnuts in "The Gluten-Free Pantry," page 35.

Flaxseed. See "The Gluten-Free Pantry," page 25.

Frangelico. A well-known hazelnut-flavored liqueur made in Italy.

Garbanzo bean flour. See Chickpea flour in "The Gluten-Free Pantry," page 30.

Garbanzo-fava flour. See Garfava flour in "The Gluten-Free Pantry," page 30.

Garfava flour. See "The Gluten-Free Pantry," page 30.

Garlic. An edible bulb composed of several sections (cloves), each covered with a papery skin. An essential ingredient in many styles of cooking.

Gelatin, unflavored. A colorless, odorless, flavorless powder used as a thickener. When dissolved in hot liquid and then cooled, it forms a jelly-like substance.

Gingerroot. A bumpy rhizome, ivory to greenish yellow in color, with a tan skin. Fresh gingerroot has a peppery, slightly sweet flavor, similar to lemon and rosemary, and a pungent aroma. Ground ginger is made from dried gingerroot. It is spicier and not as sweet or as fresh. Crystallized, or candied, ginger is made from pieces of fresh gingerroot that have been cooked in sugar syrup and coated with sugar.

Gluten. A natural protein in wheat flour that becomes elastic with the addition of moisture and kneading. Gluten traps gases produced by leaveners inside the dough and causes it to rise.

Glutinous rice flour. See Sweet rice flour in "The Gluten-Free Pantry," page 47.

Granulated sugar. A refined, crystalline, white form of sugar that is also commonly referred to as table sugar or just sugar.

Guar gum. A white, flour-like substance made from an East Indian seed high in fiber, this vegetable substance contains no gluten. It may have a laxative effect for some people. It can be substituted for xanthan gum.

Hazelnuts. See "The Gluten-Free Pantry," page 35.

Hazelnut flour (hazelnut meal). See "The Gluten-Free Pantry," page 36.

Hazelnut liqueur. The best known is Frangelico, a hazelnut-flavored liqueur made in Italy.

Hemp seed. See "The Gluten-Free Pantry," page 26.

Herbs. Plants whose stems, leaves or flowers are used as a flavoring, either dried or fresh. To substitute fresh herbs for dried, a good rule of thumb is to use three times the amount of fresh as dried. Taste and adjust the amount to suit your preference.

Honey. Sweeter than sugar, honey is available in liquid, honeycomb and creamed varieties. Use liquid honey for baking.

Italian eggplant. A miniature variety shaped like a large, plump pear, with shiny black-purple skin. Also known as baby eggplant.

Kalamata olives. See Olives, Kalamata.

Kale. A member of the cabbage family with curly pale to dark green or purple leaves. Choose green varieties for cooking.

Kasha. See "The Gluten-Free Pantry," page 21.

Lentils. See "The Gluten-Free Pantry," page 28.

Linseed. See Flaxseed in "The Gluten-Free Pantry," page 25.

Maple syrup. A very sweet, slightly thick brown liquid made by boiling the sap from North American maple trees. Use pure maple syrup, not pancake syrup, in baking.

Margarine. A solid fat derived from one or more types of vegetable oil. Do not use lower-fat margarines in baking, as they contain too much added water. See also "Lactose Intolerance," page 62.

Mesclun. A mixture of small, young, tender salad greens such as spinach, frisée, arugula, oak leaf and radicchio. Also known as salad mix, spring mix or baby greens and sold prepackaged or in bulk in the grocery produce section.

Millet. See "The Gluten-Free Pantry," page 32.

Mixed candied fruit. A mixture of orange and lemon peel, citron and glazed cherries; mixed candied peel includes orange, lemon and citron peel. Expensive citron may be replaced by candied rutabaga.

Molasses. A by-product of refining sugar, molasses is a sweet, thick, dark brown (almost black) liquid. It has a distinctive, slightly bitter flavor and is available in fancy and blackstrap varieties. Use the fancy variety for baking unless blackstrap is specified. Store in the refrigerator if used infrequently.

Montina. See "The Gluten-Free Pantry," page 33.

Nonfat dry milk. See Skim milk powder.

Nut flour (nut meal). See "The Gluten-Free Pantry," page 36.

Oats, pure uncontaminated. See "The Gluten-Free Pantry," page 37.

Oat flour, pure uncontaminated. See "The Gluten-Free Pantry," page 38.

Olive oil. Produced from pressing tree-ripened olives. Extra-virgin oil is taken from the first cold pressing; it is the finest and fruitiest, pale straw to pale green in color, with the least amount of acid, usually less than 1%. Virgin oil is taken from a subsequent pressing; it contains 2% acid and is pale yellow. Light oil comes from the last pressing; it has a mild flavor, light color and up to 3% acid. It also has a higher smoke point. Product sold as "pure olive oil" has been cleaned and filtered; it is very mild-flavored and has up to 3% acid.

Olives, green. A variety of olive that is green both before and after ripening. They are usually sold packed in olive oil or vinegar.

Olives, Kalamata. A large, flavorful variety of Greek olive, typically dark purple in color and pointed at one end.

Parsley. A biennial herb with dark green curly or flat leaves used fresh as a flavoring or garnish. It is also used dried in soups and other mixes. Substitute parsley for half the amount of a strong-flavored herb such as basil.

Pea flour. See "The Gluten-Free Pantry," page 31.

Pecan. See "The Gluten-Free Pantry," page 35.

Pecan flour (pecan meal). See "The Gluten-Free Pantry," page 36.

Pine nuts. See "The Gluten-Free Pantry," page 35.

Poppy seeds. See "The Gluten-Free Pantry," page 40.

Potato flour. See "The Gluten-Free Pantry," page 55.

Potato starch (potato starch flour). See "The Gluten-Free Pantry," page 55.

Pumpkin seeds. See "The Gluten-Free Pantry," page 40.

Quinoa. See "The Gluten-Free Pantry," page 41.

Rhubarb. A perennial plant with long, thin red- to pink-colored stalks resembling celery, and large green leaves. Only the tart-flavored stalks are used for cooking, as the leaves are poisonous. For 2 cups (500 mL) cooked rhubarb, you will need 3 cups (750 mL) chopped fresh, about 1 lb (500 g).

Raisins. Dark raisins are sun-dried Thompson seedless grapes.

Rice bran. See "The Gluten-Free Pantry," page 47.

Rice flours. See "The Gluten-Free Pantry," page 46.

Rice polish. See "The Gluten-Free Pantry," page 47.

Salba. See "The Gluten-Free Pantry," page 48.

Sesame seeds. See "The Gluten-Free Pantry," page 49.

Shortening. A solid, white flavorless fat made from vegetable sources.

Skim milk powder. The dehydrated form of fluid skim milk. Use $1/4$ cup (50 mL) skim milk powder for every 1 cup (250 mL) water.

Slurry. A mixture of a raw starch and cold liquid used for thickening.

Snow peas. An edible-pod pea with a bright green pod and small pale green seeds. Also known as Chinese snow peas and sugar peas.

Sorghum. See "The Gluten-Free Pantry," page 50.

Sour cream. A thick, smooth, tangy product made by adding bacterial cultures to pasteurized, homogenized cream containing varying amounts of butterfat. Check the label: some lower-fat and fat-free brands may contain gluten.

Sour cream, lactose-free. See "Lactose Intolerance," page 64.

Soy beverage, fortified. See "Lactose Intolerance," page 62.

Soy. See "The Gluten-Free Pantry," page 52.

Squash. An edible fruit of the gourd family; varieties are divided into winter squash and summer squash, which are not interchangeable in recipes. Winter squash has a hard shell that isn't eaten. The flesh is sweeter and stronger in flavor than that of summer squash.

Starch. See "The Gluten-Free Pantry," page 54.

Sun-dried tomatoes. Available either dry or packed in oil, sun-dried tomatoes have a dark red color, a soft chewy texture and a strong tomato flavor. Use dry, not oil-packed, sun-dried tomatoes in recipes. Use scissors to snip. Oil-packed and dry are not interchangeable in recipes.

Sunflower seeds. See "The Gluten-Free Pantry," page 59.

Sweet peppers. See Bell peppers.

Sweet potato. A tuber with orange flesh that stays moist when cooked. Not the same as a yam, although yams can substitute for sweet potatoes in recipes.

Sweet rice flour. See "The Gluten-Free Pantry," page 47.

Swiss chard. A member of the beet family with crinkly dark green leaves and silvery, red or bi-colored celery-like stalks. The leaves are prepared like spinach and have a similar tart flavor.

Tapioca. See "The Gluten-Free Pantry," page 55.

Tarragon. An herb with narrow, pointed, dark green leaves and a distinctive anise-like flavor with undertones of sage. Use fresh or dried.

Teff. See "The Gluten-Free Pantry," page 59.

Tofu. See "The Gluten-Free Pantry," page 52.

Vegetable oil. Common oils used are canola, corn, sunflower, safflower, olive, peanut, soy and walnut.

Walnuts. See "The Gluten-Free Pantry," page 35.

Whole bean flour. See "The Gluten-Free Pantry," page 31.

Wild rice. See "The Gluten-Free Pantry," page 45.

Xanthan gum. A natural carbohydrate made from a microscopic organism called *Xanthomonas campestris*, this gum is produced from the fermentation of glucose. It is used to add volume and viscosity to baked goods. As an ingredient in gluten-free baking, it gives the dough strength, allowing it to rise and preventing it from being too dense in texture. It does not mix with water, so must be combined with dry ingredients. Purchase from bulk or health food stores.

Yeast. A tiny, single-celled organism that, given moisture, food and warmth, creates gas that is trapped in bread dough, causing it to rise. Bread machine yeast (instant yeast) is added directly to the dry ingredients of bread. We use this yeast rather than active dry as it does not need to be activated in water before using. Store in the freezer in an airtight container for up to 2 years. To test for freshness, see the Technique Glossary, page 302.

Yogurt. Made by fermenting cow's milk using a bacteria culture. Plain yogurt is gluten-free, but not all flavored yogurt is.

Yogurt, lactose-free. See "Lactose Intolerance," page 63.

Zest. Strips from the outer layer of rind (colored part only) of citrus fruit. Avoid the bitter part underneath. Used for its intense flavor.

Technique Glossary

Almonds. *To blanch:* Cover almonds with boiling water and let stand, covered, for 3 to 5 minutes. Drain. Grasp the almond at one end, pressing between your thumb and index finger, and the nut will pop out of the skin. Nuts are more easily chopped or slivered while still warm from blanching. *To toast:* see Nuts.

Almond flour (almond meal). *To make:* See Nut flour. *To toast:* Spread in a 9-inch (23 cm) baking pan and bake at 350°F (180°C), stirring occasionally, for 8 minutes, or until light golden.

Baking pan. *To prepare or to grease:* Either spray the bottom and sides of the baking pan with nonstick cooking spray or brush with a pastry brush or a crumpled-up piece of waxed paper dipped in vegetable oil or shortening.

Bananas. *To mash and freeze:* Select overripe fruit, mash and package in 1 cup (250 mL) amounts in freezer containers. Freeze for up to 6 months. Defrost and warm to room temperature before using. About 2 to 3 medium bananas yield 1 cup (250 mL) mashed.

Barbecue by indirect method. To cook with the heat source coming from one or both sides of the food and not from directly beneath it.

Beat. To stir vigorously to incorporate air, using a spoon, whisk, handheld beater or electric mixer.

Blanch. To completely immerse food in boiling water and then quickly in cold water, to loosen and easily remove skin, for example.

Blend. To mix two or more ingredients together thoroughly, with a spoon or using the low speed of an electric mixer.

Bread crumbs. *To make fresh:* For best results, the GF bread should be at least 1 day old. Using the pulsing operation of a food processor or blender, process until crumbs are of the desired consistency. *To make dry:* Spread bread crumbs in a single layer on a baking sheet and bake at 350°F (180°C) for 6 to 8 minutes, shaking pan frequently, until lightly browned, crisp and dry. (Or microwave, uncovered, on High for 1 to 2 minutes, stirring every 30 seconds.) *To store:* Package in airtight containers and freeze for up to 3 months.

Cake crumbs. See Bread crumbs.

Cast-iron skillet. *To clean:* Add 2 tbsp (25 mL) salt to a dry cast-iron skillet. Rub with an old toothbrush. Keep replacing salt until it remains white. This usually requires 2 to 3 applications of salt and about 5 minutes. *To season:* Coat bottom and sides evenly with vegetable oil. Place in a 400°F (200°C) oven for 30 minutes. Turn oven off and let pan cool completely. Using a paper towel, wipe off any remaining oil.

Combine. To stir two or more ingredients together for a consistent mixture.

Cream. To combine softened fat and sugar by beating to a soft, smooth creamy consistency while trying to incorporate as much air as possible.

Cut in. To combine solid fat and flour until the fat is the size required (for example, the size of small peas or meal). Use either 2 knives or a pastry blender.

Digital instant-read thermometer. *To test meat for doneness:* Insert the metal stem of the thermometer at least 2 inches (5 cm) into the thickest part of cooked chicken, fish, pork, beef, etc. For thin cuts, it may be necessary to insert the thermometer horizontally. Meatballs can be stacked. *To test baked goods for doneness:* Insert the metal stem of the thermometer at least 2 inches (5 cm) into the thickest part of baked good. Temperature should register 200°F (100°C).

Drizzle. To slowly spoon or pour a liquid (such as frosting or melted butter) in a very fine stream over the surface of food.

Drugstore fold. *To make:* Bring the sides of parchment or foil up to meet in the center, fold over the edges, then fold the edges of the ends together. Allow room for the packets to expand, then crimp the edges.

Dust. To coat by sprinkling GF confectioner's (icing) sugar, cocoa powder or any GF flour lightly over food or a utensil.

Flaxseed. *To grind:* Place whole seeds in a coffee grinder or blender. Grind only the amount required. If necessary, store extra ground flaxseed in the refrigerator. *To crack:* Pulse in a coffee grinder, blender or food processor just long enough to break the seed coat but not long enough to grind completely.

Fold in. To combine two mixtures of different weights and textures (for example, gluten-free flours into stiffly beaten egg whites) in a way that doesn't deflate the batter. Place the lighter mixture on top of the heavier one. Use a large rubber spatula to gently cut down through the two mixtures on one side of the bowl, then gently move the spatula up the opposite side. Rotate the bowl a quarter-turn and repeat until the mixtures are thoroughly combined.

Garlic. *To peel:* Use the flat side of a sharp knife to flatten the clove of garlic. Skin can then be easily removed. *To roast:* Cut off top of head to expose clove tips. Drizzle with ¼ tsp (1 mL) olive oil and microwave on High for 70 seconds, until fork-tender. Or bake in a pie plate or baking dish at 375°F (190°C) for 15 to 20 minutes, or until fork-tender. Let cool slightly, then squeeze cloves from skins.

Glaze. To apply a thin, shiny coating to the outside of a baked, sweet or savory food to enhance the appearance and flavor.

Grease pan. See Baking pan.

Hazelnuts. *To remove skins:* Place hazelnuts in a 350°F (180°C) oven for 15 to 20 minutes. Immediately place in a clean, dry kitchen towel. With your hands, rub the nuts against the towel. Skins will be left in the towel. Be careful: hazelnuts will be very hot.

Hazelnut flour (hazelnut meal). *To make:* See Nut flour. *To toast:* Spread in a 9-inch (23 cm) baking pan and bake at 350°F (180°C), stirring occasionally, for 8 minutes, or until light golden. Let cool before using.

Herbs. *To store full stems:* Fresh-picked herbs can be stored for up to 1 week with stems standing in water. (Keep leaves out of water.) *To remove leaves:* Remove small leaves from stem by holding the top and running fingers down the stem in the opposite direction of growth. Larger leaves should be snipped off the stem using scissors. *To clean and store fresh leaves:* Rinse under cold running water and spin-dry in a lettuce spinner. If necessary, dry between layers of paper towels. Place a dry paper towel along with the clean herbs in a plastic bag in the refrigerator. Use within 2 to 3 days. Freeze or dry for longer storage. *To measure:* Pack leaves tightly into correct measure. *To snip:* After measuring, transfer to a small glass and cut using the tips of sharp kitchen shears/scissors to avoid bruising the tender leaves. *To dry:* Tie fresh-picked herbs together in small bunches and hang upside down in a well-ventilated location with low humidity and out of sunlight until the leaves are brittle and fully dry. If they turn brown (rather than stay green), the air is too hot. Once fully dried, strip leaves off the stems for storage. Store whole herbs in an airtight container in a cool, dark place for up to 1 year and crushed herbs for up to 6 months. (Dried herbs are stored in the dark to prevent the color from fading.) Before using, check herbs and discard any that have faded, lost flavor or smell old and musty. *To dry using a microwave:* Place ½ to 1 cup (125 to 250 mL) herbs between layers of paper towels. Microwave on High for 3 minutes, checking often to be sure they are not scorched. Then microwave for 10-second periods until leaves are brittle and can be pulled from stems easily. *To freeze:* Lay whole herbs in a single layer on a flat surface in the freezer for 2 to 4 hours. Leave whole and pack in plastic bags. Herbs will keep in the freezer for 2 to 3 months. Crumble frozen leaves directly into the dish. Herb leaves are also easier to chop when frozen. Use frozen leaves only for flavoring and not for garnishing, as they lose their crispness when thawed. Some herbs, such as chives, have a very weak flavor when dried, and do not freeze well, but they do grow well inside on a windowsill.

Leeks. *To clean:* Trim roots and wilted green ends. Peel off tough outer layer. Cut leeks in half lengthwise and rinse under cold running water, separating the leaves so the water gets between the layers. Trim individual leaves at the point where they start to become dark in color and coarse in texture — this will be higher up on the plant the closer you get to the center.

Mix. To combine two or more ingredients uniformly by stirring or using an electric mixer on a low speed.

Nut flour (nut meal). *To make:* Toast nuts (see Nuts), cool to room temperature and grind in a food processor or blender to desired consistency. *To make using ground nuts:* Bake at 350°F (180°C) for 6 to 8 minutes, cool to room temperature and grind finer.

Nuts. *To toast:* Spread nuts in a single layer on a baking sheet and bake at 350°F (180°C) for 6 to 8 minutes, shaking the pan frequently, until fragrant and lightly browned. (Or microwave, uncovered, on High for 1 to 2 minutes, stirring every 30 seconds.) Nuts will darken upon cooling.

Olives. *To pit:* Place olives under the flat side of a large knife; push down on knife until pit pops out.

Onions. *To caramelize:* In a nonstick frying pan, heat 1 tbsp (15 mL) oil over medium heat. Add 2 cups (500 mL) sliced or chopped onions; cook slowly until soft and caramel-colored. If necessary, add 1 tbsp (15 mL) water or white wine to prevent sticking while cooking.

Peaches. *To blanch:* See Blanch.

Pecan flour (pecan meal). *To make:* See Nut flour.

Pumpkin seeds. *To toast:* See Seeds.

Quinoa grain. *To cook:* For 1 cup (250 mL) cooked quinoa, bring to a boil ¼ cup (50 mL) quinoa and ¾ cup (175 mL) water. Reduce heat to low; cover and simmer for 18 to 20 minutes. Remove from heat. Let stand, covered, for 5 to 10 minutes, or until water is absorbed, quinoa grains have turned from white to transparent and the tiny spiral-like germ is separated.

Rice. *To cook:* See "Cooking Rice," page 46.

Sauté. To cook quickly at high temperature in a small amount of fat.

Seeds. *To toast:* There are three methods you could use: 1) Spread seeds in a single layer on a baking sheet and bake at 350°F (180°C) for 6 to 10 minutes, shaking the pan frequently, until aromatic and lightly browned; 2) Spread seeds in a single layer in a large skillet and toast over medium heat for 5 to 8 minutes, shaking pan frequently; or 3) Microwave seeds, uncovered, on High for 1 to 2 minutes, stirring every 30 seconds. Seeds will darken upon cooling.

Sesame seeds. *To toast:* See Seeds.

Skillet. *To test for correct temperature:* Sprinkle a few drops of water on the surface. If the water bounces and dances across the pan, it is ready to use.

Sunflower seeds. *To toast:* See Seeds.

Tomatoes. *To peel:* See Blanch. *To seed:* Cut fresh tomatoes in half crosswise. Squeeze to remove seeds.

Wild rice. *To cook:* See "Cooking Rice," page 46.

Yeast. *To test for freshness:* Dissolve 1 tsp (5 mL) granulated sugar in $\frac{1}{2}$ cup (125 mL) lukewarm water. Add 2 tsp (10 mL) yeast and stir gently. In 10 minutes, the mixture should have a strong yeasty smell and be foamy. If it doesn't, the yeast is too old — time to buy new yeast!

Zest. *To zest:* Use a zester, the fine side of a box grater or a small sharp knife to peel off thin strips of the colored part of the skin of citrus fruits. Be sure not to remove the bitter white pith below.

References

Case, Shelley. 2006. *Gluten-Free Diet: A Comprehensive Resource Guide*, Expanded Edition. Regina, SK: Case Nutrition Consulting.

Main, Jan. 2006. *200 Best Lactose-Free Recipes*. Toronto: Robert Rose.

Ratner, Amy. Winter 2005/2006. "Oats: Puzzle over pure oats solved." *Gluten-Free Living*.

Sullivan, Cheryl, and Kathy Rhodes. n.d. *Simply Soy: A Variety of Choices*. Frankenmuth, MI: Michigan Soybean Promotion Committee.

www.nutritiondata.com. 2006. Data from the United States Department of Agriculture.

About the Nutrient Analysis

The nutrient analysis done on the recipes in this book was derived from The Food Processor Nutrition Analysis Software, version 7.71, ESHA Research (2001).

Where necessary, data was supplemented using the following references:

1. Shelley Case, *Gluten-Free Diet: A Comprehensive Resource Guide*, Expanded Edition (Regina, SK: Case Nutrition Consulting, 2006).
2. Nutrient Data Laboratory Base for Standard Reference, Release #19 (2006). Retrieved September 29, 2006, from the USDA Agricultural Research Service website: www.nal.usda.gov/fnic/foodcomp/search/.
3. Bob's Red Mill Natural Foods. Nutritional information product search. Retrieved October 5, 2006, from www.bobsredmill.com/catalog/index.php?action=search.
4. Gluten-free oats and oat flour from Cream Hill Estates (www.creamhillestates.com). Certificate of Analysis of Pure Oats (Lasalle, QC: Silliker Canada Co., 2005). Certificate of Analysis of Oat Flour (Lasalle, QC: Silliker Canada Co., 2006).
5. Flax Council of Canada. Nutritional information product search. Retrieved October 5, 2006, from www.flaxcouncil.ca.

Recipes were evaluated as follows:

- The larger number of servings was used where there is a range.
- Where alternatives are given, the first ingredient and amount listed were used.
- Optional ingredients and ingredients that are not quantified were not included.
- Variations, including egg-free variations, were not evaluated.
- Calculations were based on imperial measures and weights.
- Nutrient values were rounded to the nearest whole number.
- Defatted soy flour, 25% reduced-sodium broth, beef stock without MSG, lactose-free skim milk, light coconut milk and brown rice flour were used, including where these ingredients are listed as soy flour, stock, beef stock, lactose-free milk, coconut milk and rice flour.
- Calculations involving meat and poultry used lean portions without skin.
- Canola oil was used where the type of fat was not specified.
- Recipes were analyzed prior to cooking.

It is important to note that the cooking method used to prepare the recipe may alter the nutrient content per serving, as may ingredient substitutions and differences among brand-name products.

Library and Archives Canada Cataloguing in Publication

Washburn, Donna
   Complete gluten-free cookbook: 150 gluten-free, lactose-free recipes,
many with egg-free variations / Donna Washburn & Heather Butt.

ISBN-13: 978-0-7788-0158-0
ISBN-10: 0-7788-0158-6

1. Gluten-free diet—Recipes. 2. Milk-free diet—Recipes.
I. Butt, Heather II. Title.

RM237.86.W373 2006   641.5'638   C2006-905908-X

Index

A

almond flour
  Apricot Almond Muffins or Loaf, 140
  Bread Sticks, 224
  Cherry Almond Biscotti, 274
  Coconut Shrimp, 92
  Linzertorte, 250
  Orange Almond Strips, 272
  Rich Dinner Rolls, 220
  Roasted Garlic Potato Bread, 192, 194
  Soda Bread, 135
  Stollen, 226
  Streusel Topping, 290
almonds, 34–35. *See also* almond flour
  Apricot Almond Muffins or Loaf,
    140
  Apricot Pecan Biscuits (variation),
    131
  Cherry Almond Biscotti, 274
  Orange Almond Strips, 272
  Streusel Topping, 290
amaranth, 19–21
amaranth flour
  Ancient Grains Bread, 176, 178
  Apricot Almond Muffins or Loaf, 140
  Biscuit Mix, 129
  Cherry Almond Biscotti, 274
  Coconut Shrimp, 92
  Fruited Barm Brack Muffins or Loaf,
    148
  Golden Harvest Muffins or Loaf, 150
  Make-Your-Own Muffin Mix, 165,
    166
  Mango and Ginger Cream Tart, 246
  Oatmeal Mincemeat Squares, 280
  Peanut Butter Cookies, 269
  Pineapple Yogurt Cupcakes, 266
  Rich Dinner Rolls, 220
  Roasted Garlic Potato Bread, 192, 194

Sourdough Loaf, 202, 204
Sourdough Savory Ciabatta, 212
Sourdough Walnut Bread, 205, 206
Streusel Topping, 290
Sunflower Flax Bread, 196, 198
Toasted Walnut Pear Muffins or Loaf,
    160
Wild Rice Cranberry Muffins or Loaf,
    162
Ancient Grains Bread, 176, 178
apple and apple juice/cider
  Apple Butter, 232
  Applesauce Apple Oatmeal Bread,
    180, 182
  Apricot Pecan Biscuits, 131
  Baked Apples, 285
  Chocolate Ginger Cake, 257
  Chocolate Pudding Cake, 260
  Cranberry Applesauce Muffins, 168
  Cranberry Walnut Quinoa Pilaf, 124
  Harvest Compote, 289
  Pumpkin Spread, 234
  Rhubarb Cobbler, 242
apricots (dried)
  Apricot Almond Muffins or Loaf, 140
  Apricot Pear Pudding, 284
  Apricot Pecan Biscuits, 131
  Baked Apples, 285
  Carrot Pecan Hermit Bars (variation),
    278
  Cranberry Walnut Quinoa Pilaf
    (variation), 124
  Fruited Barm Brack Muffins or Loaf,
    148
  Fruited Mock Pumpernickel Loaf,
    184, 186
  Golden Harvest Muffins or Loaf, 150
  Harvest Compote, 289
arrowroot, 54–55
Asian Chicken Stir-Fry, 97

R

raisins
  Banana Flaxseed Muffins (variation), 167
  Carrot Pecan Hermit Bars (variation), 278
  Cinnamon Buns, 228
  Coconut Rice, 120
  Oatmeal Raisin Cookies, 268
  Soda Bread (variation), 135
  Stollen, 226
Ratatouille, 113
Red Lentil Dosas, 134
rhubarb
  Oatmeal Rhubarb Muffins or Loaf, 154
  Rhubarb Cobbler, 242
  Rhubarb Orange Muffins or Loaf, 156
rice, 43–48. *See also* rice, brown; rice, wild; rice bran; rice flour
  Asparagus Risotto, 122
  Chicken en Papillote, 100
  Coconut Rice, 120
  cooking, 45–46
  Paella, 94
  Red Lentil Dosas, 134
  Wild Rice Latkes (variation), 118
rice, brown. *See also* brown rice flour
  Autumn Quinoa Casserole, 125
  Burritos, 104
  Cilantro Romano Pilaf, 123
  Crab and Melon Salad (variation), 80
  Cranberry Walnut Quinoa Pilaf (variation), 124
  Quinoa Salsa Salad (variation), 78
  Wild Rice Latkes, 118
  Wild Rice with Blueberries (variation), 121
rice, wild, 45
  Quinoa Salsa Salad, 78
  Sun-Dried Tomato Rice Muffins or Loaf, 158
  Wild Rice Cranberry Muffins or Loaf, 162
  Wild Rice Latkes, 118
  Wild Rice with Blueberries, 121
rice bran
  Brown Seed Dinner Rolls, 222
  Honeyed Walnut Bread, 188, 190
rice flour, 46–47
  Orange Almond Strips, 272
Rich Dinner Rolls, 220
Roasted Asparagus with Hazelnuts, 114
Roasted Garlic Dressing, 83
Roasted Garlic Potato Bread, 192, 194
Roasted Vegetables, 99
rolls, 220–23
Rubbed Roast Chicken, 96
Rum and Pecan Pie, 245

S

salads, 77–83
Salba, 48–49
  as egg substitute, 66
  Gingerbread Crumbs (variation), 238
Salmon Fillets with Lime Dijon Sauce, 90
sausage
  Black Bean Chili, 89
  Caramelized Peppers and Onions with Pasta (variation), 115
  Paella, 94
  Sausage and Leek Pizza, 87
Scallops Provençal, 91
sesame seeds, 49–50
  Bread Sticks, 224
  Brown Seed Dinner Rolls, 222
  Crispy Sesame Wafers, 70
  Halvah, 281
  Snow Pea and Red Pepper Salad, 77
Shirley's Old-Fashioned Donuts, 282
side dishes, 112–26
Six-Bean Tomato Salad, 79
Skillet Cornbread, 136
Small-Batch Make-Your-Own Muffin Mix, 166
smoothies, 71–72

Cherry Walnut Pie, 241
Chocolate Walnut Crust, 237
Cranberry Walnut Quinoa Pilaf, 124
Date Nut Muffins or Loaf, 146
Honeyed Walnut Bread, 188, 190
Pineapple Nut Muffins, 169
Rhubarb Orange Muffins or Loaf, 156
Soda Bread (variation), 135
Sourdough Walnut Bread, 205, 206
Toasted Walnut Pear Muffins or Loaf, 160
whole bean flour. *See* bean flour
wild rice. *See* rice, wild
Wild Rice Cranberry Muffins or Loaf, 162
Wild Rice Latkes, 118
Wild Rice with Blueberries, 121

Y

yogurt
Apricot Almond Muffins or Loaf, 140
Garlicky Feta Spinach Dip, 68
lactose-free, 63
Mango Smoothie (variation), 72
Pear Hazelnut Tart, 248
Pineapple Yogurt Cupcakes, 266
Rich Dinner Rolls, 220
Sun-Dried Tomato Bacon Dip, 69

Z

zucchini
Chicken en Papillote, 100
Cilantro Romano Pilaf, 123
Pasta Meatball Stew, 108
Ratatouille, 113

More Great Books
from Robert Rose

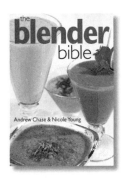

Appliance Cooking

- 125 Best Microwave Oven Recipes
  by Johanna Burkhard
- The Blender Bible
  by Andrew Chase and Nicole Young
- The Mixer Bible
  by Meredith Deeds and Carla Snyder
- The 150 Best Slow Cooker Recipes
  by Judith Finlayson
- Delicious & Dependable Slow Cooker Recipes
  by Judith Finlayson
- 125 Best Vegetarian Slow Cooker Recipes
  by Judith Finlayson
- The Healthy Slow Cooker
  by Judith Finlayson
- 125 Best Rotisserie Oven Recipes
  by Judith Finlayson
- 125 Best Food Processor Recipes
  by George Geary
- The Best Family Slow Cooker Recipes
  by Donna-Marie Pye
- The Best Convection Oven Cookbook
  by Linda Stephen
- 250 Best American Bread Machine Baking Recipes
  by Donna Washburn and Heather Butt
- 250 Best Canadian Bread Machine Baking Recipes
  by Donna Washburn and Heather Butt

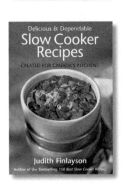

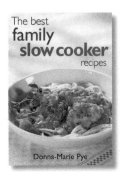

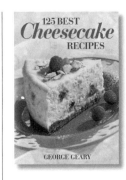

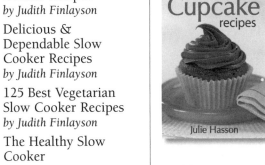

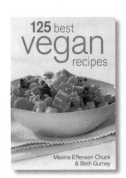

Baking

- 250 Best Cakes & Pies
  by Esther Brody
- 500 Best Cookies, Bars & Squares
  by Esther Brody
- 500 Best Muffin Recipes
  by Esther Brody
- 125 Best Cheesecake Recipes
  by George Geary
- 125 Best Chocolate Recipes
  by Julie Hasson
- 125 Best Chocolate Chip Recipes
  by Julie Hasson
- 125 Best Cupcake Recipes
  by Julie Hasson
- Complete Cake Mix Magic
  by Jill Snider

Healthy Cooking

- 125 Best Vegetarian Recipes
  by Byron Ayanoglu with contributions from Algis Kemezys
- America's Best Cookbook for Kids with Diabetes
  by Colleen Bartley
- Canada's Best Cookbook for Kids with Diabetes
  by Colleen Bartley
- The Juicing Bible
  by Pat Crocker and Susan Eagles
- The Smoothies Bible
  by Pat Crocker